Endocrinology of Cancer

Volume II

Editor

David P. Rose, M.D., Ph.D.

Professor of Human Oncology
University of Wisconsin Medical School
Associate Director for Laboratory Research
Wisconsin Clinical Cancer Center
Madison, Wisconsin

CRC PRESS, INC.
Boca Raton, Florida 33431

Library of Congress Cataloging in Publication Data

Main entry under title:

Endocrinology of cancer.

    Bibliography: p.
    Includes index.
    1. Cancer — Chemotherapy. 2. Hormone therapy.
3. Endocrine gynecology. 4. Carcinogenesis.
I. Rose, David P.
RC271.H55E54   616.9′94′061   79-498
ISBN 0-8493-5337-8
ISBN 0-8493-5338-6 pbk.

© 1979 by CRC Press, Inc.

International Standard Book Number 0-8493-5338-6

Library of Congress Card Number 79-498
Printed in the United States

PREFACE

The endocrinology of cancer has become a focal point for basic scientists and clinicians whose backgrounds lie in many different disciplines. The topic is not new; in 1889 Albert Schinzinger postulated a relationship between the ovaries and breast cancer, and seven years later George Beatson reported remissions of metastatic breast cancer in two premenopausal patients treated by bilateral oophorectomy. By the 1940s additive hormone therapy was in use, and Sir Hedley Atkins attempted to reduce the adrenal source of estrogens by subtotal adrenalectomy. With the introduction of cortisone replacement therapy, Huggins and Bergenstal were able to perform successfully bilateral adrenalectomy, a procedure to be quickly followed by pituitary ablation. Meantime, Huggins and his co-workers had also demonstrated the influence of hormones on prostatic cancer.

More recently, others have turned their attention to the endocrinology of endometrial carcinoma, both in relation to etiology and treatment with progestational agents. The application of steroid hormone receptor assays to the selection of patients for endocrine therapy provides an excellent example of how the fruits of basic research may be quickly passed on to the clinician. At present, their use is largely confined to breast cancer, but, as is discussed in this book, hormone receptor assays may also have a place in the management of endometrial cancer, malignant melanoma, and, possibly, renal cell carcinoma and prostatic cancer.

This progress in the clinical endocrinology of cancer is paralleled by extensive investigations into the role of hormones in tumor etiology. Rapid progress is being made in both the human diseases and with experimental animal tumor models. Recent interest in the nutritional aspects of cancer leans heavily on endocrinology. Collaboration between epidemiologists and endocrinologists is yielding persuasive evidence that diet plays a role in the development of some cancers by causing modifications in the hormonal milieu.

ENDOCRINOLOGY OF CANCER is an attempt to bring together basic scientists and clinicians in order to review where we are today, and the directions in which we should place our future efforts. When it appeared feasible to do so, two, in the case of breast three, chapters have been devoted to each cancer. Each time, a critical review of basic research and etiologic studies is followed by a discussion of endocrine approaches to therapy. In this way the book should prove of interest to research workers, physicians and surgeons alike. We hope that basic scientists will read the clinical discussions and find them a stimulus to their own work. Similarly, clinicians may find that the chapters concerned with laboratory-based research are of value in pointing the way to future trends in the clinical endocrinology and therapeutics of cancer.

On a personal note, I wish to thank the authors who took time to contribute to the book, Kathy Scholes, who typed several of the chapters, checked the accuracy of the references, and assisted with the proofreading, and Sandy Pearlman and Marsha Baker of CRC Press for keeping us all roughly on schedule.

David P. Rose
January 8, 1979

THE EDITOR

David P. Rose, M.D., Ph.D., is Professor of Human Oncology at the University of Wisconsin, Madison, and Associate Director for Laboratory Research of the Wisconsin Clinical Cancer Center.

Dr. Rose graduated from the University of Sheffield Medical School, England, in 1959, obtained his M.D. degree in 1964, and a Ph.D. in Chemical Pathology in 1967. From 1964 to 1969 he was lecturer in Chemical Pathology at the University of Sheffield, and subsequently moved to London to become Senior Lecturer in Human Metabolism at St. Mary's Hospital Medical School. In 1972 he took up the post of Associate Professor in Human Oncology at the University of Wisconsin, and was promoted to full Professor in 1975.

Dr. Rose's current research interests are centered on the experimental hormonal therapy of breast cancer, and the effects of chemotherapy on endocrine function.

CONTRIBUTORS

Kelly H. Clifton, Ph.D.
Professor of Human Oncology and
  Radiology
University of Wisconsin Medical
  School
Madison, Wisconsin

Alan S. Coates, M. D., F.R.A.C.P.
Specialist in Medical Oncology
New South Wales State Cancer
  Council
Randwick, New South Wales,
  Australia

P. Davies, Ph.D.
Senior Research Associate
Tenovus Institute of Cancer Research
Welsh National School of Medicine
Cardiff, Wales

Hugh L. Davis, M.D.
Associate Professor of Human
  Oncology
University of Wisconsin Medical
  School
Madison Wisconsin

Thomas E. Davis, M. D.
Assistant Professor of Human
  Oncology
Assistant Professor of Medicine
University of Wisconsin Medical
  School
Madison, Wisconsin

Richard I. Fisher, M.D.
Senior Investigator
and Attending Physician
Medicine Branch
National Cancer Institute
Bethesda, Maryland

Keith Griffiths, Ph.D.
Professor of Cancer Research
Director of Research
Tenovus Institute for Cancer Research
Welsh National School of Medicine
Cardiff, Wales

M. E. Harper, Ph.D.
Senior Research Associate
Tenovus Institute for Cancer Research
Welsh National School of Medicine
Cardiff, Wales

Clarence V. Hodges, M.D.
Professor of Surgery
Head
Division of Urology
University of Oregon Medical School
Portland, Oregon

Thomas F. Hogan, M.D.
Research Associate
Department of Human Oncology
University of Wisconsin Medical School
Madison, Wisconsin

Marc E. Lippman, M.D.
Head
Medical Breast Cancer Section
Medicine Branch
National Cancer Institute
Bethesda, Maryland

W. B. Peeling, M.A.
Consultant Urologist
Department of Urology
St. Woolos Hospital
Newport, Wales

C. G. Pierrepoint, Ph.D.
Deputy Director
Tenovus Institute for Cancer Research
Welsh National School of Medicine
Cardiff, Wales

Douglass C. Tormey, M.D., Ph.D.
Associate Professor of Human
  Oncology and Medicine
University of Wisconsin Medical School
Madison, Wisconsin

R. P. Whitehead, M.D.
Research Associate
Department of Human Oncology
University of Wisconsin Medical School
Madison, Wisconsin

TABLE OF CONTENTS

Volume I

Volume II

Chapter 1

THE ETIOLOGY AND ENDOCRINOLOGY OF PROSTATIC CANCER

K. Griffiths, P. Davies, M. E. Harper, W. B. Peeling and C. G. Pierrepoint

TABLE OF CONTENTS

I. INTRODUCTION

Prostatic cancer kills about 4000 men each year in England and Wales and is, according to the Registrar General's Statistical Review for 1968, the fourth commonest cause of death from malignant diseases in men. There has been a tendency to ignore these facts, partially because prostatic cancer is confined to men in their later years and, therefore, lacks the drama of cancer of the breast and bronchus which can strike down people in their prime, but also because it occurs in what is, to the general public, a hidden and little known anatomical site inaccessible to all but the most meticulous clinician. The prostate is not a reality to patients and their relatives because it cannot be seen or felt like the breast, and it has no obvious function like the lungs or gastrointestinal tract, so they accept its presence as a mysterious influence that is likely to make micturition difficult when they get old. To many men, the inconvenience of prostatism is merely a barometer of their advancing years, which to them is a fact of life, like gray hair and decreasing exercise tolerance, and clinicians have similarly accepted that pathological changes giving rise to benign or malignant tumors in the prostate are also features of aging. This assumption tends to divert attention away from possible influences related to prostatic tumors that may occur in the early life of males when certain events would 'prime' the prostate and determine its eventual benign or malignant career. Therefore, any study concerning prostatic tumors should attempt to define clearly its relationship to benign or malignant diseases for, as discussed later, these are separate *clinical* conditions that arise in different parts of the prostate and are likely to have different biological characteristics. It is often difficult to do this, particularly in laboratory work, because the cornerstone of all endocrinological studies concerning the prostate has been the fact that its growth, maintenance, and functional activity are largely dependent upon androgenic hormones secreted by the testes and this concept has been applied towards the treatment of both malignant and benign prostatic tumor. The relation between testicular function and the prostate was known 200 years ago when John Hunter[1] reported that castration was followed by a decrease in size of the prostate gland.

The use of orchidectomy to treat prostatic hypertrophy followed some years later.[2,3] Administration of diethylstilbestrol as a form of antiandrogen therapy for carcinoma of the prostate then developed from the classical laboratory experiments of Dr. Charles Huggins and colleagues,[4-6] which established the concept that prostatic cancer cells also retained some degree of hormone dependence similar to that of the normal gland, so that antiandrogen therapy, either by estrogen administration or orchidectomy, is now the usual form of primary treatment for this disease. This is effective for the majority of patients, since up to 80% can be expected to improve clinically following treatment,[7] although the extent and duration of response is unpredictable, and many of these men will eventually relapse. It would seem that relapse occurs because only a proportion of the neoplastic cells are hormone responsive, and progression of the disease results from the autonomous nature of the remainder which eventually kill the patient. It is obvious that the precise effects of endocrine therapy in the management of prostatic cancer are yet to be clearly established. Furthermore, the endocrine factors concerned with the etiology of the condition are also little understood. It may well be that the hormonal role in the pathogenesis of prostatic cancer is more permissive rather than inciting, for present knowledge offers few leads that relate hormonal factors with the initiation of neoplasia. Investigations related to endocrine status and etiology have, until now, been directed to the influence of androgens on prostate growth, the androgen-estrogen balance, the effect of estrogens on prostatic biochemistry and to pituitary, adrenal, and testicular activity. Certainly the clinical behavior of prostatic cancer tends to reflect androgen stimulation. The disease has not been reported in the prepubertally castrated male and evidence, currently available, tends to suggest a definite role for certain hormones in the promotion of abnormal prostatic growth.

A. Certain Aspects of the Pathogenesis and Epidemiology of Prostatic Cancer

Until quite recently, much of the research into the pathogenesis of prostatic cancer has tended to be dominated by the observation of Franks[8,9] that sclerotic atrophy, attributable to elevated estrogen levels, was probably a precancerous condition. Sommers[10] supported this observation and Liavag[11] has since described the association between atrophic prostatic epithelium and the presence of latent carcinoma. The concept that prostatic cancer originated from atrophic tissue, possibly resulting from a decreasing testicular activity of the aging male, has not, however, received much support from subsequent investigations of recent years.

A possible relationship between benign prostatic hypertrophy and carcinoma of the gland has also been a subject of controversy for many years. The high frequency of nodular hyperplasia in prostatic cancer, observed at autopsy,[10] led Armenian and colleagues[12] to reassess the concept that patients with benign prostatic hypertrophy might be at risk of developing malignant disease later in life. They reported a study in which 300 patients who had been treated for benign prostatic hypertrophy and a similar number of age-matched controls were traced until death. There was a 3.7 times higher death rate from prostatic cancer in the group that had a previous history of prostatic disease. They concluded from their data that hypertrophy may be a direct cause or an intermediate stage between causative factors and carcinoma. This information, together with the observation that the highest mortality rates for benign prostatic hypertrophy and cancer of the prostate are found in Iceland and the developed European countries[13]—with the lowest rate for both conditions in Asian countries such as the Philippines, Singapore, and Japan—tends to favor the concept that the two conditions are related. The possibility that hyperplasia constitutes a premalignant condition cannot be summarily dismissed, although it would be reasonable to expect to find carcinoma and nodular hyperplasia in the same prostatic tissue since prostatic enlargement is common in the aging male. There are indeed, numerous reports of latent carcinoma associated with clinical benign hypertrophy of the prostate.[14,15]

The consensus among urologists has generally been, however, that prostatic cancer is not directly related to hypertrophy and this is supported by another report, that of Greenwald et al.,[16] who studied 800 patients with benign prostatic hypertrophy, again with matched controls. They were followed for 11 years and the results indicated that a similar proportion from both groups subsequently developed prostatic cancer. This study, therefore, offers support for the general opinion that benign prostatic hypertrophy and carcinoma are independent conditions and suggests that research must be based on the concept that the diseases have separate etiologies. Although some of the problems associated with this type of study have been discussed,[17,18] the importance of investigations into the natural history of prostatic disease and of careful epidemiological studies cannot be overemphasized.

In trying to understand the relationship between the etiology of prostatic carcinoma and the endocrine status of patients with the disease, many investigators have attempted to define the effective hormonal disturbance from detailed study of various histological changes observed in tissue removed from the patients. Considerable controversy has arisen in recent years[19] concerning the precancerous changes observed in resected prostatic tissue. Franks has consistently maintained[8,9,20] that a particular type of focal atrophy could be recognized, often associated with lymphocytic infiltration and fibrosis of the periepithelial stroma, which could be considered precancerous. Definite areas of proliferation which develop from this atrophic epithelium have a pattern closely resembling the structure of small acinar carcinoma. McNeal, with a newly developed concept on the anatomy of the prostate gland in which function, morphology, and pathology have been effectively interrelated,[19,21] has clearly indicated[19] that he is diametrically opposed to such views.

An appreciation of McNeal's thoughts on the development of prostatic cancer in

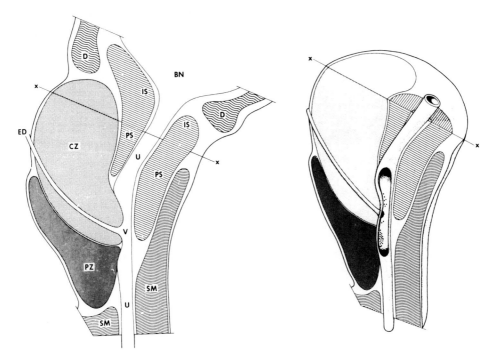

FIGURE 1.   Diagrammatic representation of the anatomy of the prostate with reference to the McNeil concept. CZ, central zone; PZ, peripheral zone; V, verumontanum; U, urethra, ED, ejaculatory duct; PS, preprostatic sphincter; IS, internal sphincter; SM, external sphincter muscle; BN, bladder neck; D, detrusor muscle. (Drawn after discussion with Blacklock, N. J., in *Scientific Foundation of Urology*, Vol. 2, Williams, D. I. and Chisholm, G. D., Eds., W. Heinemann Medical Books, New York, 1976, 113. With permission.)

certain regions of the human prostate is best seen in relation to his concept of the anatomy of the gland. This is considered a composite of three distinct, separate glandular structures within a single capsule,[22] with two, the central zone and the peripheral zone, forming the "true functional prostate" (Figure 1). The third glandular structure is the periurethral gland, a series of small ducts opening into the upper segment of the urethra which lies above the upper end of the verumontanum and extends upwards to the bladder neck. This upper section of the urethra is enclosed in a cylinder of muscle tissue that functions as a urinary preprostatic sphincter.

Unlike the fully developed glandular tissue of the central and peripheral zones, the periurethral glands are small, simple structures which are not thought to contribute to the production of seminal fluid. In McNeal's view, the periurethral zone of the prostate is a distinct element in its own right, and previous descriptions that considered it to be part of the true prostate are not correct. Lowsley[23] from a study of the anatomy of the fetal prostate also considered that these glands were not part of the prostate proper. The central and peripheral zones of the prostate generally undergo progressive but slow atrophy with increasing age, although with considerable individual variation such that older prostates can display glandular morphology comparable to that seen in glands from younger men.[22] McNeal, however, decribed an age-related increase in atypical hyperplasia, diffuse or multifocal proliferation of ductal and epithelial tissue from "persistently active glandular tissue"—premalignant changes which were considered closely associatcd with prostatic carcinoma. A high incidence of carcinoma was found in the presence of atypical hyperplasia and, on occasion, continuity between this premalignant tissue and the origin of small foci of invasive cancer. Focal atrophy, described by Franks, was considered a condition secondary, not to aging, but to inflammation.[19]

In McNeal's study[22] 170 small carcinomas (under 3 mm in diameter) were identified in the 415 prostates examined, and, of these, 148 were in the peripheral zone and none were found in the periurethral gland. This glandular structure McNeal considers the unique site of origin of benign nodular hypertrophy. Blacklock,[24] in an excellent review of the surgical anatomy of the human prostate, strongly supported the views of McNeal from his own personal observations. Koppel and colleagues,[25] in a retrospective study of the pathology of prostatic tissue, have also indicated that diffuse hyperplasia was found significantly more often in tissue from prostatic cancer patients than in controls and they considered the relevance of their observations in relation to pathogenesis of the disease.

It is interesting that Reischauer in 1925[26] also believed that the earliest hyperplastic changes occurred in the fibromuscular stroma, with associated epithelial proliferation, in the preprostatic urethral sphincter.

Small, asymptomatic latent carcinoma is relatively common in prostatic tissue, particularly in regions of the peripheral zone furthermost from the urethra. Their prognosis poses a difficult question and the proportion becoming clinically manifest has yet to be decided. The latent period before these tumors become more aggressive is probably considerable and the biochemical or endocrine conditions which promote the changes are unknown. Some believe[27,28] that these microscopic foci of differentiated carcinoma rarely become clinically manifest. The time course is certainly difficult to establish and extensive neoplastic change could occur in these peripheral sites of the carcinoma, with early capsular involvement and spread of the disease outside of the prostate taking place before clinical signs were evident. From an autopsy series in which the occurrence of prostatic carcinoma in routinely sectioned glands was considered,[29] the frequency, on *routine* sectioning at 75 years of age, was found to be the same as that from *serial* sections taken at 55, and it was suggested, therefore, that there was at least a 20-year lapse between the initial development of the neoplasm and its clinical manifestation.

Promotion of prostatic neoplasia may, therefore, be dependent upon an abnormal endocrine status of certain older males. At present, there are little data on even epidemiological characteristics relating to this disease. It was always hoped that factors which might reflect the hormonal status of a man prior to cancer development would assist in delineating a high-risk group, but studies of demographic features such as age, socioeconomic class, marital status, sex drive, etc. of subjects who presented with prostatic carcinoma have generally failed to consistently produce significant differences from control groups.[30-32] Often conflicting reports in the literature have tended to cloud the issues. Kessler,[33] for example, failed to demonstrate increased prostatic cancer mortality among diabetics despite Lea's observation[34] that a high death rate from prostatic cancer relates to a high mortality from diabetes. Although Bourke and Griffin[35] reported a high incidence of diabetes mellitus in an English population with benign prostatic hyperplasia, Greenwald et al.[16] were unable to support the claim.

It is obvious, however, from studies of migrating populations that environmental and socioeconomic factors can influence the etiology of prostatic cancer.[36] Death from the disease is rare in the Japanese as it is in other oriental populations, yet this rate increases to nearly half that of the indigenous American for those Japanese that become domiciled in the U.S. A number of epidemiological studies have been concerned with prostatic cancer in the Japanese male.[37,38] It is interesting that the low incidence of prostatic cancer in Japan relates only to clinical cancer, since autopsy data show

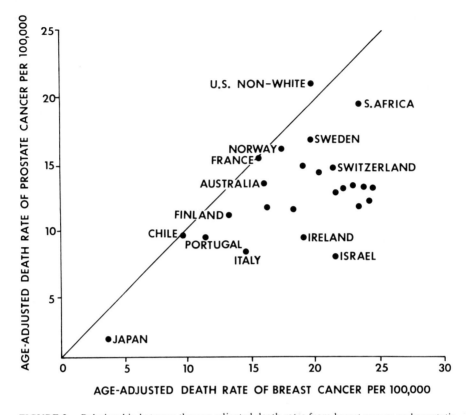

FIGURE 2.   Relationship between the age-adjusted death rates from breast cancer and prostatic cancer. (Data from Wynder, E. L., Mabuchi, K., and Whilmore, W. F., *Cancer (Philadelphia)*, 28, 344, 1971. With permission.)

that latent carcinoma is present as much as in Caucasians of corresponding ages. Investigations have obviously been directed to the evaluation of endocrine differences between Japanese and Caucasian men in the different age groups. Urinary 17-ketosteroid excretion was lower in the former, although the plasma concentrations of testosterone and cortisol were similar in the two populations.[39,40] In a more recent study, Okamoto and colleagues[41] suggested that there was a unique pattern of testosterone metabolism in the Japanese male.

Detailed, careful epidemiological studies must now be of great potential value in assessing those biological factors that may be concerned with the etiology of prostatic cancer. The high mortality rate from this disease in the American Negro compared to the Negro from Africa[36] directs attention to the environment. The positive correlation between prostatic cancer and carcinoma of the breast[36] (Figure 2) suggests a common type of etiological background for these hormone-related cancers, and, obviously, intensive investigation into the endocrinology of the normal and diseased prostate gland could eventually provide a valuable guide to possible cause. The following sections outline some of these investigations.

II. HORMONES AND AGING

Clinical data indicate that carcinoma of the prostate in man is, to some extent, functionally dependent upon androgenic stimulation, yet the role of the various C_{19}-steroids circulating in the blood and formed within the prostate, in the etiology of the disease, remains obscure. Considerable interest has been directed to the changes in plasma steroids that are associated with aging in man and to the relative activity of the endocrine glands that play a part in the regulation of prostatic growth and function.

Testosterone must be considered to be the most important plasma androgen and the concentration, of its free, nonprotein-bound form, is generally accepted as a reasonable indicator of androgenic status. This status does not depend solely upon plasma testosterone, however, but also relates to other C_{19}-steroids, many of which can achieve relatively high levels in blood, steroids such as androstenediol (androst-5-ene-3β,17β-diol), androstenedione, DHA (dehydroepiandrosterone), and DHA sulfate. The interrelationship between these various plasma steroids and their glands of origin must be considered in any discussion concerned with the endocrinology of prostatic disease and the influence of aging on androgen balance. The recent development of radioimmunoassay for hormone analysis has allowed the sensitive and precise measurement of various steroids and protein hormones present in plasma and has contributed greatly to our understanding of the problem.

A. Endogeneous Steroid Hormone Levels in Plasma

It was interesting that, although prostatic disease occurs at a time when it is generally accepted that testicular function is declining, Kent and Acone reported[42] that the plasma concentration of testosterone in the human male is maintained at a relatively constant level from the age of 20 to the ninth decade. This resulted, however, from a decrease in the metabolic clearance rate of the hormone rather than a sustained ability of the testis to continue with its active synthesis and secretion. In contrast, Vermeulen and colleagues[43] observed that the testosterone concentration decreased after the sixth decade, although individual differences were large (Table 1).

In this respect, Vermeulen also showed that sex hormone binding globulin (SHBG) retained a constant binding capacity until about the fifth decade, when a gradual increase occurred until, at the age of 80, its value was approximately twice that found in young men. The free, nonprotein-bound, testosterone fraction, which represents about 2% of the total testosterone concentration in the younger man, decreases to 1.75% in the fifth decade and to 1.25% in the eighth. Therefore, although the total testosterone concentration in plasma at the age of 80 is one third of that at 25, the "active" free fraction represents only one sixth. This is referred to again in a later section.

Androgen levels in plasma may, therefore, decrease with aging in certain individuals, particularly after the sixth decade, and data from other groups tend to support this concept,[44-47] although in most of these investigations the significance of the differences found between the various age groups studied has not been sufficiently convincing to indicate that this is a general phenomenon. For most studies, control subjects can only be men without clinically manifest prostatic disease, and it would seem that more detailed studies of individual subjects will be necessary. On the other hand, plasma estradiol-17β concentration was found to increase with age in the healthy, apparently normal, adult male[44,48] (Table 1), thereby supporting the concept that changes in the androgen-estrogen balance in elderly men may be implicated the the etiology of prostatic disease.

Little is known about the physiological importance of estrogens in the male. It has been established that the testis secretes estradiol-17β and estrone,[49-51] although its contribution to the plasma estrogen levels is small. Any involvement of the adrenal cortex is, however, negligible and the major proportion of plasma estrogen in the male origi-

TABLE 1

Steroid Hormone Concentrations in Plasma of Men

Plasma steroid concentration

	Testosterone (ng/ml)			Estradiol-17β (pg/ml)			5α-Dihydrotestosterone (pg/ml)
Age groups	Kent and Arone[42]	Vermeulen et al.[43]	Harper*	Pirke and Doerr[44]	Kley et al.[48]	Bartsch et al.[65]	Mahoudeau et al.[45]
20—30	6.35	6.16	5.77				640
30—40	5.60	6.34	5.54	16.6	19.7	16.2	640
40—50	4.70	6.40	5.62				810
50—60	5.90	5.82	5.43				650
60—70	5.90	4.62	4.45				610
70—80	6.50	3.73	—	25.6	28.7	24.2	460
>80	2.80	2.45	—				640

* Accumulated data from the Tenovus Institute for Cancer Research.

nates from the peripheral aromatization of such steroids as androstenedione and testosterone,[52,53] the former being synthesized and secreted by the adrenal cortex.[54] Little quantitative data are available on estrogen production from C_{19}-steroids in relation to aging or in patients with carcinoma or hypertrophy of the prostate, although it has been reported,[55] that increased peripheral aromatization occurs in the elderly man, which could, therefore, account for the increased plasma estrogen/androgen ratio.

Kley and colleagues[56] assessed the effect of age on the responsiveness of the adrenal cortex and testis to trophic stimulation. In 12 younger men (19 to 40 years old) and 12 elderly subjects (60 to 86 years old), adrenocorticotrophic hormone (ACTH) administration resulted in a 250% rise in plasma cortisol in both age groups, with a concomitant 100% rise in plasma estrone in the former and a 75% rise in the older group. There was little or no effect of ACTH on plasma estradiol-17β levels. In the younger group, HCG (human chorionic gonadotropin) administration increased plasma concentration of estrone (122%) and also that of estradiol-17β (250%), whereas in the older group it was considered there was a relative, decreased response to HCG, with increases of plasma estrone and estradiol-17β of 103% and 150%, respectively. Again, whether this response reflects direct secretion of estrogen or that of a prehormone is difficult to determine from such experiments. Doerr and Pirke[57] showed a similar response of the testis to HCG and also studied the suppression of testicular secretory activity with fluoxymesterone. Both studies show, however, that the ability to respond to exogenous gonadotropin is preserved despite aging and loss of libido.

B. Steroid Hormone Binding Proteins

In assessing the androgenicity of the plasma steroids, it is important to recognize that many of them are bound to plasma proteins[58] which would, therefore, modulate their activity. Testosterone, 5α-dihydrotestosterone (5α-DHT, 17β-hydroxy-5α-androstan-3-one), the 5α-androstanediols, androstenediol, and, also, estradiol-17β, bind with high affinity but low capacity—and with some degree of stereospecificity—to a β-globulin referred to as the sex hormone binding globulin. A 17β-hydroxyl group and a 3-keto-function appear necessary for binding.[61] Albumin will also bind steroids but with such low affinity that it has little physiological significance. There is also good evidence that the free, nonprotein-bound hormone represents the biologically active component[62] so the distribution of the various plasma steroids between free and bound states must, therefore, be taken into account when considering potential androgenicity and

TABLE 2

Sex Hormone Binding Globulin in Man

Age groups	Sex hormone binding globulin (SHBG) binding capacity	Ref.
Normal males		
20—50	5.2×10^{-8}M	63
70—85	8.9×10^{-8}M	
20—40	2.28×10^{-8}M	65
50—85	3.62×10^{-8}M	
22—44	2.85×10^{-8}M	64
45—64	4.66×10^{-8}M	
20—50	4.3×10^{-8}M	66
50—90	7.8×10^{-8}M	
Prostatic cancer		
54—80	3.89×10^{-8}M	64
50—85	4.00×10^{-8}M	65
Prostatic hypertrophy		
62—97	4.07×10^{-8}M	64
Estrogen-treated carcinoma	14.0×10^{-8}M	64

also the concentration of SHBG. In this respect, therefore, the observed increase in SHBG with advancing age[44,63-66] (Table 2) together with the consequent decrease in plasma free testosterone levels[43,67] must be relevant when considering the effect of this androgen on the aging prostate. The increase in SHBG would seem to have a lesser effect on the plasma concentration of free estradiol. In the case of this hormone, there was an approximate 7% decrease in the level of the free steroid with advancing age, which emphasizes again the change in the "biologically active" estrogen and androgen balance in the elderly male (Table 3). It is generally assumed that the increase in the concentration of SHBG results from the increase in plasma estrogens.

Little is known about the biochemical processes concerned with the transfer of plasma steroid into the target cells, but obviously the relationship between plasma-bound and free concentrations must play a role. Farnsworth considered this relationship as a possible mechanism for controlling the intracellular accumulation of steroid within the prostate,[68] and it has been generally accepted that only free steroid is available to androgen-dependent tissues.[69] Lasnitzki and Franklin[70] showed with explants of rat prostate in culture that serum containing SHBG inhibited the entry of testosterone into the cells. Similar results from human prostatic tissue have also been obtained.[71] A more intensive investigation into the factors which control steroid entry would be valuable, and it would seem reasonable that intracellular receptor concentration, steroid metabolism in the prostate, and possibly certain protein hormones such as prolactin may be concerned. There has also been some speculation that SHBG, with steroid attached, may bind to the plasma membrane to mediate steroid transfer into the cell or, indeed, that SHBG could pass through the membrane. There are many studies to develop on this aspect of prostatic endocrinology, some of which may be of particular relevance to chemotherapy.

C. Steroid Metabolism in the Prostate: 5α-Dihydrotestosterone and the 5α-Androstanediols: Biological Effects

In normal men, more than 90% of the testosterone produced each day, which is

TABLE 3

Free Nonprotein Bound Steroids in Plasma from Men

Age groups	Plasma-free steroid (% Total)			Conc-free steroid in plasma			
	Testosterone	5α-DHT	Estradiol-17β	Testosterone (pq/mℓ)	5α-DHT (pq/mℓ)	Estradiol-17β (pq/mℓ)	Ref.
22—61	2.24	1.17	2.49	122	5.78	0.42	67
67—93	1.65	0.83	2.31	69	4.29	0.56	
20—50	2.08						63
50—70	1.68						
70—90	1.36						

approximately 5 to 10 mg, is secreted by the testes with a relatively small contribution from the adrenal cortex,[72] although, as discussed later, this is significant in the estrogen-treated or orchidectomized man. Furthermore, there is now considerable evidence to indicate that 5α-dihydrotestosterone, rather than testosterone, is the active, intracellular hormone in the prostate gland and other accessory sex organs.[73-76] The formation in vitro of 5α-dihydrotestosterone from testosterone by tissue preparations from human benign hypertrophic prostate was originally demonstrated in the now classical experiments of Farnsworth and Brown.[77] Further studies, with human and animal tissues, undertaken by Farnsworth and a number of other groups including our own,[68,78-80] confirmed and expanded these original findings. Many other metabolites of testosterone are formed in vitro, especially 5α-androstane-3α,17β-diol and 5α-androstane-3β,-17β-diol, and it was of interest when [7α-³H]testosterone was infused as a bolus into the cephalic vein of human subjects undergoing Millin retropubic prostatectomy for benign prostatic hypertrophy that the radioactive steroids isolated from the prostatic adenoma, removed about 30 min later, showed a similar pattern of testosterone metabolism to that observed in vitro,[80,81] with 5-α-dihydrotestosterone appearing as the major radioactive product (Table 4). Androstanediols were also formed, together with androsterone, epiandrosterone, 5-α-androstanedione, androstenedione, and, in some of the experiments in vivo,[81] epitestosterone (17α-hydroxyandrost-4-en-3-one) and 5α-androstane-3β,17α-diol (Figure 3). It is possible of course that radiometabolites formed by systemic interconversion may be localized in the prostate and this has been discussed by Voigt and colleagues who have performed similar studies in vivo.[82]

It would also appear that metabolites of testosterone other than 5α-dihydrotestosterone may have specific roles to play within the target tissue. Baulieu, Lasnitzki and Robel[83,84] showed that certain 5α-androstanediols, as well as 5α-dihydrotestosterone, stimulated cell division and induced epithelial hyperplasia and secretory activity in cultured explants of rat prostate. The investigations of Farnsworth[68,85] suggest that 5α-androstane-3α,17β-diol may influence the steroid-sensitive, cation-dependent ATP-ase in human prostatic tissue directing attention to effects of steroids on prostatic biochemistry other than intranuclear processes. Our own studies[86-88] have indicated that certain of the 5α-androstanediols stimulate a semipurified prostatic DNA polymerase (DNA nucleotidyltransferase, E.C. 2.7.7.7) and DNA-dependent RNA polymerase (nucleoside triphosphate-RNA nucleotidyltransferase E.C. 2.7.7.6). It seems then that testosterone and certain of its metabolites are concerned in the control of prostatic growth and function, and interconversion of these steroids within the gland may provide a delicate regulatory mechanism for the various glandular processes. Imbalance of this mechanism could be considered a possible factor which might contribute to prostatic dysfunction. The part played by other hormones such as prolactin, growth

TABLE 4

Radioactive Steroids Isolated in Human Prostatic Tissue after In Vivo Infusion of 50μCi [7α-³H]Testosterone, [7α-³H]Androstenedione, or [7α-³H]Dehydroepiandrosterone (DHA) Sulfate

% Total radioactivity associated with the carrier steroids

	Testosterone infusion Patient no.					Androstenedione infusion Patient no.				DHA sulfate infusion Patient no.		
	31	32	33	34	35	23	24	38	39	36	37	40
Testosterone	9.2	12.8	7.4	3.2	3.1	6.6	18.1	4.7	2.0	2.2	2.0	0.2
5α-Dihydrotestosterone	51.2	74.2	72.4	66.4	55.5	2.5	6.6	11.0	16.2	1.0	4.9	0.2
Androsterone	8.7	5.9	11.1	6.2	14.3	8.8	9.2	24.3	24.6	3.2	7.5	0.3
Epiandrosterone	5.5	2.3	1.9	3.4	6.2	39.7	47.3	29.4	17.7	2.2	6.6	0.3
5α-Androstanedione	1.5	1.2	1.3	4.5	5.2	—	0	13.8	1.9	0	0	0
Androstenedione	6.8	0.9	0.4	5.6	2.8	35.2	0	10.9	14.2	1.6	3.1	0.3
5α-Androstane-3β,17β-diol	8.9	2.7	2.4	5.6	5.5	3.1	10.6	2.8	9.2	0	0	0
5α-Androstane-3α,17β-diol	5.7	—	2.9	5.1	7.4	3.8	8.3	2.6	13.8	0	0	0
DHA	—	—	—	—	—	—	—	—	—	2.2	2.6	8.8
DHA sulfate	—	—	—	—	—	—	—	—	—	89.4	72.9	89.8

Note: Dashes indicate steroid was not investigated in these experiments.

Data from Harper, M. E., Pike, A., Peeling, W. B., and Griffiths, K., *J. Endocrinol.*, 60, 117, 1974.

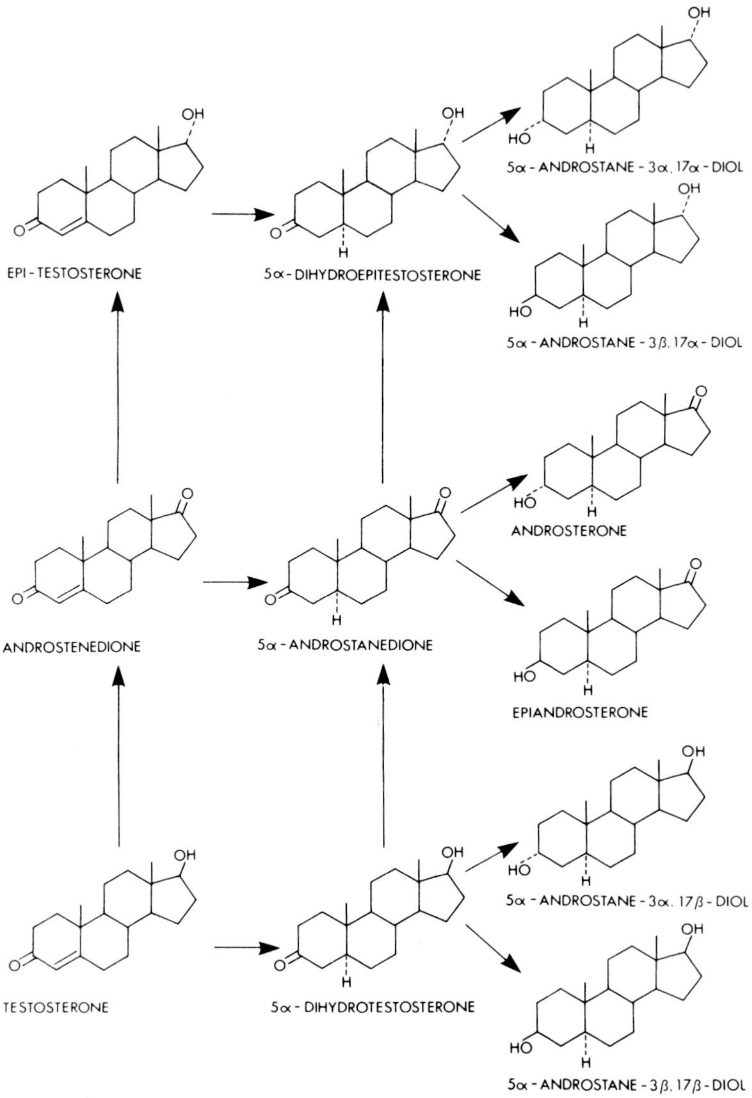

FIGURE 3.   Testosterone metabolism by the prostate.

hormone, insulin, and estrogens in influencing this metabolic pattern is not yet understood. It must be accepted that at present the androgenic role of the androstanediols is not particularly clear. Possibly, knowledge of their concentrations in plasma could well provide an index of prostatic activity with regard to testosterone metabolism. Furthermore, 5α-androstane-3α,17β-diol may have a function in inhibiting FSH and LH secretion by the pituitary,[89,90] but whether it has any androgenic function per se must be doubtful. Although this diol is apparently an effective androgen[91] in that its administration to castrated rats increased the ventral prostate weight to the same extent as that achieved with 5α-dihydrotestosterone (Table 5), the elegant, extensive investigations of Voigt and colleagues[71,82,92] effectively demonstrated that the major product in hypertrophic prostates of man, injected with [^{3}H]5α-androstane-3α,17β-diol, was 5α-dihydrotestosterone. Less 5α-dihydrotestosterone was found after administration of [^{3}H]5α-androstane-3β-17β-diol. It is difficult, therefore, to distinguish the andro-

TABLE 5

Weight of the Ventral Prostate After Steroid Administration to Castrated, Mature Rats

Treatment[a]	Ventral prostate wt (mg/100 g body wt) Mean ± SD
Sesame oil	16.5 ± 6.4
Testosterone	50.4 ± 2.8
Epitestosterone	22.3 ± 3.6
5α-Dihydrotestosterone	67.5 ± 1.8
5α-Androstane-3α,17β-diol	66.4 ± 10.2
5α-Androstane-3β,17β-diol	20.1 ± 3.3
5β-Androstane-3α,17β-diol	22.1 ± 10.4

[a] Rats were treated daily with 100 μg steroid/100 g
body weight, s.c., for 7 days, starting on the day or
orchidectomy. Steroids were given in sesame oil.

Data from Eik-Nes, K. B., *Vitam. Horm. (N. Y.)*, 33,
193, 1975.

genic effects of these diols from those of 5α-dihydrotestosterone to which they are
both metabolized. In the rat, however, if conversion of the 5α-androstane-3β,-17β-diol
to 5α-dihydrotestosterone does not occur,[93] then the biological effects observed by
Robel et al.[94] and Schmidt et al.[95] must be attributed to that diol for which there may
exist an equally specific receptor.

Early studies from the Tenovus Institute[88] provided evidence that 5α-androstane-
3α,17α-diol may play a role in controlling RNA synthesis in the canine prostate. Evidence for a specific receptor for this diol has been found by Evans and Pierrepoint[96]
as well as for 5α-dihydrotestosterone,[97] although only the former steroid was able to
maintain the histological integrity of the tissue in organ culture.[98] Epitestosterone and
5α-dihydroepitestosterone were only partially successful in maintaining epithelial
height, while secretory activity was not preserved. Testosterone and 5α-dihydrotestos-
terone were entirely unsuccessful in this respect and induced a marked stromal reaction. Obviously, a greater insight is needed into the effects of the various metabolites
of testosterone of prostatic biochemistry.

D. Metabolic Activity of the Prostate Gland

Although an assessment of prostatic activity could be made from enzyme studies on
tissue preparations in vitro, it has always been believed that the measurement of the
various prostatic metabolites of testosterone in biological fluids could ultimately provide the best index of prostatic function, or dysfunction, in vivo. Specific radioimmunoassay for the different 5α-androstanediols are only now being developed, however,
and at present, little is known about the levels of these steroids in plasma.

Vermeulen and colleagues[43,99] studied the effect of advancing age on testosterone
metabolism along the lines previously followed by Mauvais-Jarvis and colleagues[100-
102] when investigating androgen metabolism in normal women. Decreased formation
of the 5α-androstanediols in the older man was reported, with an increase in the 5β/
5α-metabolite ratio, a metabolic pattern observed in men on estrogen therapy[63] and in
hypogonadism.[103] Since estrogen treatment decreases the concentration of plasma 5α-
androstane-3α,17β-diol, which is related to the level of the free plasma testosterone

fraction, Vermeulen et al.[43] suggested that these metabolic changes observed with advancing age were consistent with a decreased metabolism of testosterone in target tissues such as the prostate.

It was established by Ito and Horton[104] that in the normal male plasma 5α-dihydrotestosterone is derived principally from testosterone. Its blood-production rate is approximately 400 μg/day,[105] half of which originates from peripheral conversion of plasma testosterone, 20% from androstenedione,[106,107] and a smaller amount is synthesized and secreted by the testes.[108] Although it is unlikely that metabolism of androgens within the prostate makes a significant contribution to the levels of 5α-dihydrotestosterone in the circulation, the observations by Mahoudeau et al.[45] are of interest, for they found that blood taken from the prostatic capsular veins of nine men undergoing open prostatectomy for benign hyperplasia contained slightly higher levels of this steroid than systemic venous blood. It is, however, difficult to accept that prostatic capsular venous blood is likely to reflect accurately the character of blood leaving the true prostate, for there is a most complex plexus in this region communicating with the dorsal vein of the penis, the base of the bladder, and, possibly, the epididymis and testicular venous drainage through the deferential vein. Mahoudeau and colleagues recognized this limitation. They also found that there was no difference in the ratio of 5α-dihydrotestosterone to testosterone in the plasma of 29 men with benign prostatic hyperplasia when compared with age-matched controls whose prostates were observed to be normal at operation for other disorders. Furthermore, no significant reduction of this ratio was found in peripheral venous blood after removal of a prostatic adenoma. This contrasts with the findings of Berberia and his colleagues[109] who reported an increased ratio of 5α-dihydrotestosterone to testosterone in the plasma of men with benign prostatic hypertrophy and, after resection of the prostatic tissue, the level of 5α-dihydrotestosterone decreased. These data, therefore, suggest that a prostatic adenoma can contribute substantially to plasma 5α-dihydrotestosterone levels, and the impressive superfusion studies of Giorgi et al.[110] certainly indicated that 5α-dihydrotestosterone was released from prostatic tissue. Whether the normal prostate contributes in a similar manner remains to be demonstrated. Further study is also required to consider the effect of prostatectomy on pituitary hormone secretion, since it would seem from experimental evidence, to be discussed later, that certain protein hormones such as prolactin may influence prostatic activity.[111,112]

It is also important to establish whether 5α-dihydrotestosterone secreted by the normal prostate gland reflects the loss of an excess of metabolite formed, but not associated with androgen receptor,[113] or the release of 5α-dihydrotestosterone previously bound to nuclear chromatin after translocation of steroid-receptor complex from cytoplasm to nucleus. The biochemical mechanisms which regulate prostatic metabolism of testosterone and the processes which govern 5α-dihydrotestosterone action and release are, as yet, poorly understood, and, consequently, the value of measuring plasma 5α-dihydrotestosterone levels for the assessment of prostatic activity requires careful consideration. In contrast to testosterone, the plasma concentration of total 5α-dihydrotestosterone was shown not to decrease with advancing age when Pirke and Doerr[114] analyzed plasma from men between the ages of 22 to 61 and 69 to 93. Mahoudeau et al.[45] also failed to show a significant decrease in 5α-dihydrotestosterone levels with increasing age (Table 1), although conflicting data from the laboratory of Chisholm[115] did indicate a lower concentration in elderly men.

A significant 26% decrease in free, nonprotein-bound 5α-dihydrotestosterone in plasma was reported[114] however, although this was still smaller than the 46% decrease in free testosterone levels found between the different age groups (Table 3), and the close relationship between the concentration of the two steroids—with a 5α-dihydrotestosterone to testosterone ratio of approximately 0.1—suggests that plasma 5α-dihydrotestosterone concentration is essentially a function of plasma testosterone levels.[116]

It is difficult to know whether plasma levels of 5α-dihydrotestosterone accurately reflect 5α-reductase activity in that, although the prostate may secrete this steroid, further intracellular metabolism to the 5α-androstanediols obviously affects the amount released. It was shown in the rat, however, by Shimazaki et al.[117] that castration decreased 5α-reductase activity and, furthermore, by Moore and Wilson,[118] that administration of testosterone increased the activity of the enzyme. It is noteworthy that opposite effects of these endocrine manipulations have been reported for the 5α-reductase of the adrenal cortex[119] and pituitary glands.[120]

Animal model systems can often be used to investigate human disease and Eik-Nes[91] has recently considered the relevance of the prostatic secretion of 5α-dihydrotestosterone in the isolated organ from the dog when substances that affect the metabolic activity of the prostate enter the gland through the arteries under controlled blood flow[121] and then are removed, together with their metabolites, in the venous drainage. The effect of end-product inhibition of enzymatic activity is, therefore, avoided. The perfused canine prostate concentrates androgens, and perfused testosterone is rapidly metabolized to 5α-dihydrotestosterone and other metabolites.[122] Furthermore, analytical data on affluent and effluent blood indicated that the prostate secreted 5α-dihydrotestosterone. It is important, however, when studying the endocrinology of the canine prostate, that extrapolation to man should be undertaken with considerable care. The tendency of the dog, like man, to develop an age-related hypertrophy of the prostate[123,124] and, less commonly, neoplasia,[125,126] recommends this animal for special consideration in its own right. From such a study in the Tenovus Institute, the presence of a specific receptor protein for 5α-androstane-3α,17α-diol,[96] which stimulated RNA polymerase activity in an isolated in vitro system,[127,128] suggested that there are probably basic underlying differences in the endocrine control of prostatic function between the two species. More intensive research on the dog may make more evident the endocrine changes that initiate or accompany prostatic dysfunction in this species.

III. HORMONAL STATUS OF PATIENTS WITH PROSTATIC DYSFUNCTION

It seems reasonable that in the search for the biochemical or endocrine abnormality that could be concerned in the etiology of prostatic cancer, a detailed study of the hormone levels in plasma and tissue from patients with this disease could provide valuable information. The generally accepted experimental approach has been that a comprehensive knowledge of hormone action and steroid metabolism in diseased prostatic tissue and in tissue from normal elderly men, together with information on the hormonal status of patients from whom tissue was removed, could provide the necessary background that would lead to a greater understanding and possibly control of prostatic disease.

It has been realized, however, that there is yet little evidence to indicate that plasma hormones are actively concerned in prostatic carcinogenesis, although few would deny that the differentiated carcinoma is usually androgen dependent. Certainly, conventional therapy has involved reducing plasma testosterone or possibly inhibiting its action within the prostatic cell. It is possible, therefore, that activation of latent carcinoma and promotion of its early growth involve hormone intervention, although, as described earlier, opinions tend to differ as to whether a reduced androgenic status with associated prostatic atrophy[8,20] or prostatic hyperplasia[19,22] precedes neoplasia.

In relation to this, hormone profiles in patients with benign prostatic hypertrophy have also been determined, again in comparison with the asymptomatic "normal" male, and it is not yet understood whether any endocrine disturbances associated with hypertrophy similarly influence to any extent the development of neoplasia.

A. Plasma Hormones and Prostatic Disease

It has been accepted for many years that estrogens may play an important role in male reproductive physiology and there has long been speculation that changes in the androgen-estrogen balance may be implicated in the etiology of prostatic disease.[129-132] Prostatic hyperplasia and the synergism occurring between androgens and estrogens in promoting the growth of the prostate and seminal vesicles have been discussed often.[133]

Since the plasma concentration of estradiol-17β has been shown to increase with age in the apparently normal, healthy adult male, a report from Brandes et al.[134] on ultrastructural studies of prostatic adenomas, indicating androgen stimulation with an overriding estrogenic effect, would, therefore, seem reasonable; others[135] have confirmed this observation. Studies with experimental animals also indicate that estrogens can induce prostatic enlargement, although the relevance of the effect in relation to the pathogenesis of prostatic hypertrophy in man must be viewed with some degree of caution. Spontaneous prostatic adenocarcinoma has been described in rodents,[136,137] but benign hypertrophy can only be induced by hormone manipulation. For example, Burrows and Kennaway[138] produced urinary obstruction by the application of estrogenic material to the skin of mice and Fingerhut and Veenema[139] reported growth of the periurethral glands and the prostate in mice after prolonged treatment with diethylstilbestrol. Although these classical studies are interesting, experimental prostatic enlargement does not have the histological fibrotic characteristics typical of the human benign tumor, and use of rodents as a model system may be limited.[140]

Studies from our own laboratories[141] have been concerned with the plasma levels of testosterone, androstenedione, estradiol-17β, FSH, LH, and prolactin in patients with prostatic cancer, with benign prostatic hyperplasia, and in controlled hospitalized patients without symptomatic or clinical prostatic disease (Table 6). With the exception of prolactin, no significant difference was noted in the concentration of these hormones between any of these groups. The mean plasma prolactin concentration was significantly lower in the patients with benign hyperplasia than in those with malignant disease. Asano[142] earlier, using a bioassay, claimed an increased urinary excretion of prolactin in patients with prostatic cancer; and Bartsch et al.[65] have also reported an elevated prolactin level in 15% of such patients with carcinoma.

The data on plasma C_{19}-steroid levels agree well with results of Moon and Flocks.[143] Previously, Isurugi[144] had found no evidence of an elevated testosterone production rate in patients with prostatic carcinoma. Although Gandy and Peterson[145] described an elevated peripheral concentration of androstenedione in six patients with prostatic carcinoma, implicating the adrenal cortex, in our study of 23 patients (Table 6), no such elevation was detected. Bartsch et al.[65] also confirmed that plasma levels of testosterone, 5α-dihydrotestosterone, estrone, and estradiol-17β, in patients with prostatic cancer, did not differ from those of a control group of similar age. Despite the implication, therefore, that estradiol-17β may be concerned in the pathogenesis of prostatic hyperplasia, these investigations[65,141] indicated that all the patients studied had similar levels of plasma estradiol-17β. This agreed with earlier reports of Marmorston et al.[146] on estrogen measurements in urine from a similar group of patients.

It may well be, however, that the relevant time to study such estrogen changes is many years earlier, long before the disease is manifest. Alternatively, differences may exist between concentrations of unbound estradiol-17β in the various groups. It is also

TABLE 6

Plasma Hormone Concentrations in Patients With and Without Prostatic Disease[a]

		Testosterone (ng/ml)	Androstenedione (ng/ml)	Estradiol (pg/ml)	LH (mIU/ml)	FSH (mIU/ml)	Prolactin (mamp/ml)
Control groups of patients without prostatic disease	Mean value	6.4	0.56	40	7.0	14.0	16.4
	SEM	0.5	0.06	1.2	1.4	4.2	4.0
	n	35	32	34	35	31	35
Patients with benign prostatic hypertrophy	Mean value	5.9	0.59	41.7	11.1	6.6	9.5[a]
	SEM	0.4	0.06	1.6	1.5	1.4	1.4
	n	41	27	41	41	37	41
Patients with prostatic carcinoma	Mean value	5.45	0.70	38.5	8.2	6.9	19.0
	SEM	0.46	0.11	1.6	1.6	2.5	3.5
	n	33	23	30	33	31	32

[a]   Benign v. prostatic carcinoma P≥0.01, n = number of patients, SEM = standard error of the mean.

possible that biochemical changes within the cell, resulting in an increased sensitivity and responsiveness to the normal hormone levels, could lead to abnormal growth.

Despite experimental work in animals that suggested that pituitary hormones may influence prostatic growth and function,[146,147,149] there have been few studies on plasma protein hormones and prostatic cancer. Hypophysectomy, for example, in dog[150] and rat[151] produces a more marked prostatic atrophy than does castration. Administration of growth hormone (GH) and ACTH to hypophysectomized-castrated rats stimulated prostatic growth,[151] whereas LH, FSH, and prolactin were without effect. Synergism of hormonal effects was evident, for simultaneous administration of prolactin and ACTH to castrated rats produced greater prostatic growth than ACTH alone.[152] A more marked increase in fructose and citric acid content of the prostate of hypophysectomized-castrated rats was found after prolactin and testosterone administration than after testosterone alone,[153] the effect being mainly on the dorsolateral lobe of the gland. GH was generally found to complement the effects of prolactin and testosterone on prostatic weight.[154]

Although plasma hormones may not be actively concerned in prostatic carcinogenesis, a permissive role should not be overlooked and a particular endocrine milieu could influence tumor dissemination. Similarly, tumor spread may affect the secretion of stress-related hormones such as ACTH, cortisol, GH, and prolactin. A study was established in the U.K. to examine in considerable detail possible interrelationships between these plasma hormones and a variety of clinical parameters. The investigation was established under the auspices of the British Prostate Study Group consisting of urologists from various clinics in the country in association with the Tenovus Institute for Cancer Research. Patients who presented for treatment in different clinics were selected, assessed, and classified in a standardized manner, according to their primary tumor grade and metastatic status, and a profile of plasma hormone levels was determined prior to and during therapy. Possible differences in hormone concentrations between these particular groups were investigated by using a multivariate-statistical-analysis technique developed at the Institute by Wilson and Tan.[155] Canonical variate analysis was used to determine if group separation could be achieved and to establish the contribution of the various hormones in discriminating between the various patient populations. Particular attention was given to ensure consistent assay performance over a prolonged period, and special quality control schemes were devised for use in the Institute's hormone assay laboratories.[156-158]

Concentrations of testosterone, estradiol-17β, FSH, LH, prolactin, and GH in the plasma of patients classified according to their primary tumor staging (modified UICC[159] classification) are given in Table 7. Mean values, together with standard deviations, are shown and the wide variation between individuals in each group is evident. No significant differences were found between these groups using the standard Student's 't' test. Table 8 shows the mean values for plasma hormones of patients with (M1) and without (M0) evidence of metastases. Again, no significant differences were found. Use of canonical variate analysis led to discrimination between various groups.[160] Figure 4 illustrates the separation of the variate-group means when patients with T3- and T4-stage tumors were analyzed against those with T0, T1, and T2 tumors, the circles representing the 95% confidence regions for these means. The principal components resulting in the separation of the groups were estradiol-17β and GH, which contributed 21% and 27% of the variance, respectively. GH levels were lower in patients with more advanced tumors, which is interesting since this hormone is released in response to stress, a response that might be expected in this group of patients. When plasma hormone concentrations of patients classified into two groups, based on the presence and absence of clinically evident metastases, were subjected to multivariate analysis, separation of the variate means was obtained (Figure 5) with age (62%) and

TABLE 7

Plasma Hormone Concentrations of Patients with Prostatic Carcinoma Separated According to UICC Classification of Their Primary Tumors

Classification group (No. of patients)		Age (years)	Plasma hormone concentrations					
			T ng/ml	E₂ pg/ml	LH mIU/ml	FSH mIU/ml	GH μU/ml	Prolactin mμ/ml
T₀ category	mean	71	4.5	29.5	6.4	15.5	3.1	0.1
(n = 24)	SD	9.04	1.48	17.65	5.33	13.05	3.72	0.13
T₁ category	mean	68	4.6	27.0	6.7	16.9	1.6	0.1
(n = 14)	SD	7.07	2.03	9.33	5.28	16.07	2.44	0.09
T₂ category	mean	71	4.4	29.4	5.4	15.1	3.8	0.1
(n = 31)	SD	9.23	1.60	11.06	4.13	14.03	7.06	0.10
T₃ category	mean	70	4.1	26.2	8.2	16.8	2.5	0.1
(n = 73)	SD	7.86	1.53	12.11	8.09	17.27	3.49	0.11
T₄ category	mean	68	3.7	24.5	6.5	14.6	3.7	0.1
(n = 21)	SD	7.43	1.31	7.53	7.15	22.46	4.85	0.11

Note: T refers to testosterone, E_2 to estradiol-17β, S.D. to standard deviation and n to the number of patients.

GH (31%) the principal discriminating components. GH means were higher in the group with metastases, and the biochemistry of sommatomedin in relation to metastatic spread of tumor to bone may well be of interest. FSH levels were found to be significantly different in patients with benign and malignant disease when using this form of analysis (Figure 6; Table 7). Whether concentrations of these various hormones are in any way related to the histological grading of the tumor in individual patients is currently being studied by the Prostate Study Group. This may be relevant when assessing the possible feedback control by tumor metabolites. Androgen metabolism of the more differentiated prostatic tumors probably differs from those which are anaplastic,[161] and other studies from the Institute in the field of carcinoma of the breast indicated that the more highly differentiated primary breast tumor rarely lacks estradiol-17β receptors.[162]

It is obvious, however, that further studies along these lines, on the interrelationship of hormone levels and various clinical parameters, can do much to elucidate the role of the endocrine factors in the pathogenesis of prostatic cancer.

The relationship of prolactin to prostatic disease requires detailed investigation. The effect on plasma prolactin levels of the increasing estradiol to testosterone ratio in the elderly male has not been fully documented and is under review by the British Prostate Study Group, but the well-established stimulatory effect of estrogen on prolactin release[141,163,164] may be concerned in disturbing prostatic biochemistry. Preliminary studies have produced evidence that prolactin in vitro, may increase the effectiveness of testosterone action on the prostate by increasing the uptake of the steroid by the gland,[68,111,147] but the precise mechanism by which prolactin affects the prostate remains uncertain. Results from this Institute[165] clearly indicate that administration of CB154 (2-bromo-α-ergocryptine, Sandoz Ltd.), an inhibitor of prolactin secretion,[166] to male rats for periods up to 30 days, failed to affect the weights of the accessory sex glands despite the decrease in plasma prolactin concentration to an undetectable level.

B. Endogenous Steroid Levels in Prostatic Tissue

It has been suggested that changes in steroid metabolic activity of the prostate may

TABLE 8

Plasma Hormone Concentrations of Patients with Prostatic Carcinoma with and without Clinical Evidence of Metastases and of Patients with Benign Prostatic Hyperplasia

Group		Age (years)	Plasma hormone concentrations					
			T ng/ml	E$_2$ pg/ml	LH mIU/ml	FSH mIU/ml	GH μU/ml	Prolactin mμ/ml
Patients without metastases MO	mean	70	4.3	25.9	7.8	18.5	2.4	0.10
(n = 78)	SD	8.15	1.38	9.46	7.80	19.70	4.71	0.11
Patients with metastases M1	mean	70	4.1	27.1	6.0	13.0	3.4	0.10
(n = 74)	SD	8.28	1.74	13.34	5.05	13.00	4.28	0.12
Benign prostatic hyperplasia	mean	68	4.3	30.9	7.3	7.7	2.6	0.14
(n = 72)	SD	8.3	1.9	12.0	5.6	7.7	2.2	0.08
Significant differences	MO	V Benign	NS	0.01	NS	0.001	NS	NS
	M1	V Benign	NS	NS	NS	0.001	NS	NS

Note: T refers to testosterone; E$_2$ to estradiol-17β; n to numbers of patients; SD to standard deviation and NS to not significant.

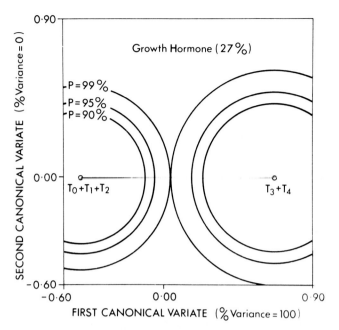

FIGURE 4.   Separation of variate group means by canonical variate
analysis. The circles represent the confidence regions for each of the
tumor categories; the centres of the circle represent the variate group
means. GH contributes 27% of the variance in the separation between
group T0, T1, T2 and T3, T4.

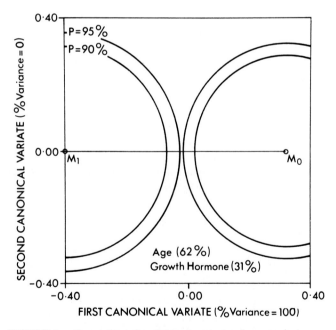

FIGURE 5.   Separation of variate groups means by canonical variate analysis. As with Figure 4, group separation was achieved and
GH and age contributed to the discrimination of the M1 and M0
groups.

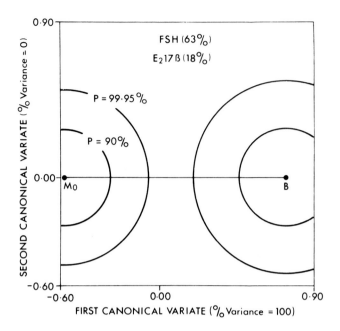

FIGURE 6.   Separation of variate groups means by canonical variate analysis. FSH contributes to the separation of the benign and M0 carcinoma categories.

be responsible for the pathogenesis of the diseased state. Whether prolactin affects metabolism or uptake of testosterone by benign or malignant tumor cells remains to be elucidated. Interesting in this respect, however, was the observation of Siiteri and Wilson[167] that the endogenous concentration of 5α-dihydrotestosterone in benign prostatic adenomas was five times greater (Table 9) than in normal post-mortem prostatic tissue and, furthermore, that there was a higher level of the "active androgen" in the periurethral region of the prostate compared with the other zones.

The known effect of 5α-dihydrotestosterone on prostatic growth,[91] its mitogenic effect on explants of rat ventral prostate in culture,[72,73] the marked rise in its concentration in prostatic tissue from men over 60 years of age, and the correlation between canine prostatic size and 5α-dihydrotestosterone content[168] prompted Siiteri and Wilson[167] to suggest that increased production and accumulation of this steroid in the periurethral area of the prostate results in abnormal tissue growth.

From our own work on the development of high-resolution, selected ion-monitoring procedures for the analysis of steroid levels in biological tissues,[169] endogenous concentrations of testosterone, 5α-dihydrotestosterone, 5α-androstane-3α,17β-diol, and 5α-androstane-3β,17β-diol were also determined[170] in a limited number of benign prostatic adenomas (Table 9). The levels of testosterone and 5α-dihydrotestosterone were similar to those reported by Siiteri and Wilson, and the 5α-androstanediol concentrations to results recently obtained by Geller et al.[171] for 'total androstanediol' levels. The data of Geller et al. suggest that the increased level of 5α-dihydrotestosterone results from a decreased 3-hydroxysteroid oxidoreductase activity which is responsible for converting 5α-dihydrotestosterone to the diols. Certainly it appears that there is no difference in the 5α-reductase activity of normal and abnormal tissue.[167] The levels of endogenous steroids in prostatic carcinoma will be awaited with particular interest.

It has been mentioned that the canine prostate is also prone to hyperplastic change with age. Early reports from Ofner[79] and ourselves[78] recorded the formation, in the

TABLE 9

Endogenous Steroid Concentrations in Prostatic Tissue

	Endogenous steroid concentrations (ng/g tissue)			Investigation (method)
	5α-Dihydrotestosterone	Testosterone	5α-Androstanediols	
Normal prostate	2.1 ± 0.32 (0.78—2.9)	—	10.2 ± 2.4 (total diols)	Geller et al.[171] (RIA)
	1.3 ± 0.5 (0.3—1.9)	0.9 ± 0.3 (0.1—4.6)	—	Siiteri and Wilson[167] (double isotope dilution)
Hypertrophic prostate	5.6 ± 0.93 (3.1—9.2)	—	2.3 ± 0.3(total diols)	Geller et al.[171](RIA)
	6.0 ± 1.0	0.9 ± 0.2	—	Siiteri and Wilson[167] (double isotope dilution)
	12.7 ± 7.1	1.7 ± 0.6	1.06 ± 0.23 [5α-androstane-3α,17β-diol] 0.53 ± 0.12 [5α-androstane-3β,17=-diol]	Millington et al.[170] GC—MS

Note: RIA refers to radioimmunoassay and GC-MS to gas chromatography - mass spectrometry.

canine prostate, of 5α-dihydrotestosterone and the various androstanediols, and it was recognized that the formation of the latter group of steroids may regulate the intracellular concentration of 5α-dihydrotestosterone. An interesting experiment of Jacobi and Wilson[172] involved the incubation of 5α-dihydrotestosterone with microsomal preparations from homogenates of 31 dog prostates, from 1 to 15 g weight. 5α-Androstane-3α,17β-diol formation correlated with the size of the gland, which is also known to relate to age, and it was suggested that androstanediol biosynthesis may be a limiting factor in controlling prostatic growth in the dog with excessive synthesis inducing prostatic hyperplasia. The 3α,17β-diol does increase prostatic size in the dog[118] although it was originally considered to act only after conversion to 5α-dihydrotestosterone.[173] As previously stated, the androstanediols could have a unique role in mediating androgen action[133,174] and may be worthy of further study.

IV. ESTROGENS, PROLACTIN, AND THE TESTICULAR-PROSTATIC AXIS

Obviously, androgen uptake by the prostate is influenced by the nature of the steroid in the blood and the capacity of the cell to retain and metabolize it. The potential effects, both direct and indirect, of the higher estrogen to androgen ratio in the older man on androgen action and prostatic metabolism, require more careful consideration.

The well-established elevation of plasma prolactin after estrogen administration has been discussed. The effects in the elderly man of increasing plasma SHBG levels, probably-induced by estrogen, have been considered. SHBG levels control the plasma concentration of free C_{19}-steroid and estradiol-17β and, therefore, steroid availability to the hormone-dependent tissues. Voigt and his co-workers[64] recently confirmed the age dependency of SHBG binding capacity and produced data suggesting that a lower

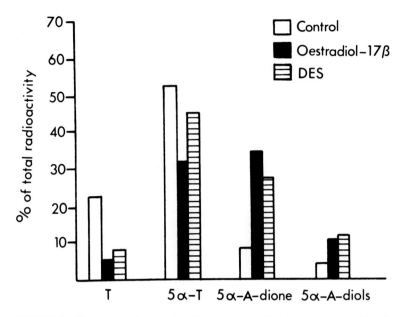

FIGURE 7.   Rat prostate incubated with testosterone. Animals were treated for 10 days (100 µg/day, i.m.) with either estradiol-17β or diethylstilbestrol. Controls received sesame oil only. Prostatic tissue (1 g) was incubated with [7α-³H]testosterone in Krebs Ringer bicarbonate-glucose for 1 hr at 37°C. Reaction products were analyzed as described.[181] T, testosterone; 5αT, 5α-dihydrotestosterone; 5α-A-dione, 5α-androstane-3,17-dione; 5α-A-diols, 5α-androstanediols.

SHBG binding capacity occurred in benign and malignant disease of the prostate. However, the increased level of SHBG determined in these patients after subsequent estrogen therapy clearly did not indicate any disturbance in SHBG regulation, and subsequent studies[65] failed to confirm this interesting observation.

The increased concentration of plasma free estradiol-17β in the elderly man could exert a more direct action on the prostate and the observed effect of estradiol-17β, in increasing the uptake of testosterone by the lateral lobe of the rat prostate is noteworthy.[175] Superfusion studies of Giorgi et al.[176] also indicate that estrogens increased the entry of testosterone into the prostate. On the other hand, in other experimental systems[177,178] there was a decreased formation of 5α-dihydrotestosterone in the presence of estrogen. Shimazaki and colleagues had also shown previously that estrogen reduced 5α-reductase activity,[179] but had no effect[117] on the reduction in vitro of 5α-dihydrotestosterone to 5α-androstane-3α,17β-diol.

Circulating estradiol-17β as well as prolactin[68,111,147] could, therefore, influence the endogenous C_{19}-steroid content of the aging and, also, dysfunctional prostate, although the experimental data available as yet suggest that there is no concomitant, increased formation of 5α-dihydrotestosterone. Indeed, treatment of dogs with estradiol-17β for 30 days produced a marked change in the C_{19}-steroid metabolic pattern of the prostate, with an apparent stimulus to the "oxidative pathway" (Figure 3), resulting in the formation of the less androgenic androstenedione and 5α-androstanedione at the expense of testosterone and 5α-dihydrotestosterone.[180] Our own experiments[78] also produced evidence that estrogen administration increased the rate at which testosterone was metabolized by canine prostatic tissue, an effect subsequently confirmed in rat prostatic tissue.[181] These latter studies (Figure 7) demonstrated that daily administration of estradiol-17β or diethylstilbestrol in vivo for 10 days markedly af-

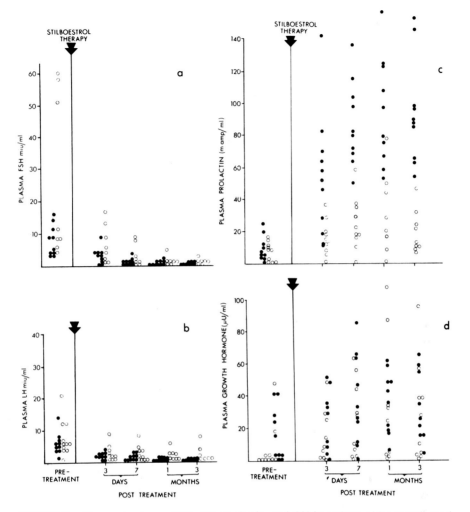

FIGURE 8. Changes in plasma FSH, LH, Prolactin, and GH in patients with prostatic carcinoma before and after treatment with diethylstilbestrol (O) 1 mg t.d.s. or (•) Honvan, 100 mg
b.d. (Data from Harper, M. E., Peeling, W. B., Cowley, T., Brownsey, B. G., Phillips, M. E.
A., Groom, G., Fahmy, D. R., and Griffiths, K., *Acta Endocrinol. (Copenhagen),* 81, 409, 1976.
With permission.)

fected testosterone metabolism in vitro by prostatic tissue, with a decreased formation
of 5α-dihydrotestosterone and a corresponding increase in the synthesis of the 5α-an-
drostanediols and 5α-androstanedione.

A. Estrogen and the Pituitary-Testicular Axis

Although there is evidence that estrogens directly influence the prostate gland, it has
generally been considered that the principal antiandrogenic effect of estrogen therapy
in the treatment of prostatic carcinoma is exercised, indirectly, on prostatic tissue, via
the pituitary, reducing testosterone secretion by suppression of LH release. Such an
effect has been observed in patients with prostatic cancer[182] and Figure 8 illustrates
the marked changes in gonadotropin levels in treated patients from our own studies.[141]
There is little evidence that the changing estrogen to androgen balance can influence
circulating FSH or LH, or that changes in gonadotropin levels relate to prostatic dysfunction, except as mentioned earlier; accumulated analytical data indicated a differ-

ence in the levels of FSH between patients with benign and malignant tumors (Figure 6). Geller et al.[183] have reported a decreased LH reserve in elderly men with benign disease, although no age-matched controls were used in this study. Such studies to assess the relationship of circulating hormone levels to prostatic disease have generally involved only single plasma determinations and must, therefore, be considered with caution. Frequent sampling during a 24-hr period would be more effective, as would an investigation in depth into the chronobiology of the endocrine aspects of prostatic disease. This is illustrated by the observed change in LH secretion with age. Detailed studies of plasma LH levels during the complete 24-hr sleep-wake cycle of males up to the age of 45 clearly demonstrated an augmented LH secretion during the sleep period in late prepubertal and early pubertal males[184,185] which contrasted with the low LH secretion before puberty. The elevated LH secretory activity during sleep marks the onset of clinical puberty,[186] a process in which secretion of androgens by the adrenal cortex may be concerned.[187,188] Advancing sexual maturity is characterized by episodic secretion of LH during the wake periods until the mean LH levels during these times are the same as those found in sleep.[189]

Similar detailed studies of LH secretion with advancing age are not yet available, although there are investigations which indicate that plasma LH levels from single analyses increase each decade from the age of 40,[190] but data on prostatic disease are limited. Urinary-protein-hormone analysis with sampling through a 24-hr period to assess secretion in relation to prostatic cancer may be worth considering.

An increase in plasma LH with advancing age[190] may well reflect a decreasing capacity of the testis to synthesize testosterone,[43] although this cannot be considered hypogonadism, since in both young and elderly men, HCG administration has been shown to increase both plasma testosterone[57,191-194] and estrogens.[36,194] The absolute response was a little less in the elderly, but the ability to respond was preserved. Others[195,196] were unable to show a change in basal levels of FSH and LH with advancing age, although the capacity of the pituitary to respond to administered LH-RH tended to decrease with age. Similar decreased FSH and LH "responses" to LH-RH stimulation have been described[99,197] in relation to male senescence, although in every study marked pituitary stimulation was observed. The relative "unresponsiveness" may well result from the effect of the increasing plasma estradiol-17β in older men on LH-RH action. Our own studies,[198-200] which illustrate the effect of estradiol-17β on pituitary responsiveness to LH-RH in dog and man, are shown in Figure 9.

In considering the changing testicular-prostatic axis with age, the suggested direct inhibitory action of estrogen on the testis[201-203] should also be considered. Estrogen administration in vivo was subsequently shown to have affected the testicular synthesis of testosterone in vitro[78,181,204] in particular by decreasing the activity of both the 17β-hydroxysteroid dehydrogenase and 17α-pregnen-C-17,20-steroid lyase.

The concept of a direct inhibitory action of estrogens on testicular synthesis of testosterone has long been controversial,[205] but experimental data tend to support both an immediate direct action together with a delayed, less sensitive effect at the pituitary level. It is clear, however, that advancing age is accompanied by changes in testicular function reflected by decreased spermatogenesis, although whether this results from reduced steroid synthesis remains to be elucidated. Possibly the number of Leydig cells decreases with age,[206] or they are relatively less sensitive to gonadotropins, but the interrelationship of these testicular changes to prostatic disease is not clear. Little is also known about the effect of aging on the Sertoli cells and their function.

B. Prolactin and the Testicular-Prostatic Axis

Prolactin secretion by the pituitary is controlled by prolactin inhibiting factor re-

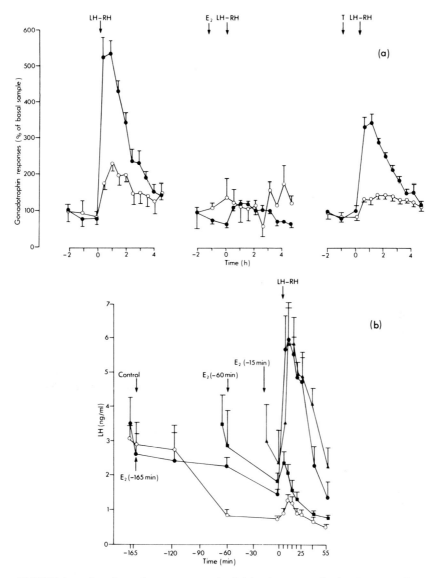

FIGURE 9.   Gonadotropin responses to luteinizing hormone-releasing hormone (LH-RH): (a) in man, with no pretreatment and after injection (i.m.) of either estradiol-17β (E₂) or testosterone (T) 2 hr. previously. FHS (○) and LH (●) concentrations in plasma were normalized by expressing as a fraction of the average within an experiment for each man. Mean values (± S.E.M., n = 5 men) were calculated and are presented as percentages of the initial, basal sample. (Data from Cole, E. N., Llewelyn, H., Link, J., and Boyns, A. R., *J. Endocrinol.*, 63, 251, 1974. With permission.) (b) in male beagle dogs (6) given 50 μg E₂ in 0.15 M NaCl or vehicle alone. Experiments were over 4 weeks and were randomized. Blood was collected before and after administration of 5 μg LH-RH 15, 60, or 165 min after E₂ injection. Vertical lines indicate ± S.E.M. (Data from Jones, G. E. and Boyns, A. R., *J. Endocrinol.*, 61, 123, 1974, and 68, 475, 1976. With permission.)

leased by the hypothalamus and, currently, considered by some to be dopamine.[207] There is at present little information on the effect of aging on prolactin secretion, although there was a comparable prolactin response when TRH was administered to groups of males of different ages,[208] an observation subsequently confirmed by Yamaji et al.,[209] who also stated that aging per se did not appear to be associated with alterations in the basal prolactin secretion or the pituitary reserve of the hormone. Data are needed, however, on the episodic secretion of prolactin in the older man and the changes in the circadian rhythms of prolactin output with advancing years. In view of this episodic secretion of prolactin, only regular and frequent sampling over a more extended time period will provide the necessary reliable assessment of the physiological role of prolactin in the elderly man.

Evidence is now accumulating that prolactin plays a physiological role, probably synergistically with LH, in regulating testicular activity. Specific binding of ^{125}I-ovine prolactin to rat testicular membrane preparations has been reported,[210] and the work of Hafiez and colleagues[211,212] suggests that prolactin and LH are required to maintain normal plasma levels of testosterone in hypophysectomized rats. Although in some species, there is a parallel fluctuation in the plasma levels of testosterone and LH,[213] indicating that testosterone production is predominantly under LH control: such a relationship was not found in man.[214] Studies from our own laboratories[111] on the interrelationship between gonadotropins, testosterone, and prolactin in six normal young men over a 24-hr period showed a correlation between prolactin and testosterone in three subjects. Rubin et al.[215] also reported a correlation between peripheral levels of prolactin and testosterone and have previously observed[216] from nocturnal episodic-hormone-secretion studies that the testosterone peak was preceded by an elevation in prolactin.

Administration to normal men of sulpiride, a dopaminergic antagonist promoting prolactin synthesis, followed by HCG-stimulation of testicular activity, also resulted in an enhanced testosterone output in the presence of hyperprolactinemia.[217] In contrast, however, hyperprolactinemia in the female has an antigonadotropic effect[218,219] and furthermore, transplantation of prolactin-producing tumors to male rats led to testicular atrophy.[220] Our own investigation of infertility in the human male[221] indicated that hypoprolactemia was also related to infertility, the general interpretation probably being that physiological prolactin levels are required for normal testicular function.

A role for prolactin in the endocrine control of the testis seems clear, therefore, although the mechanism by which this regulation is effected still requires clarification. Possible underlying abnormalities in prolactin secretion that could lead to prostatic dysfunction in the elderly man demand further investigation and the physiological control by the testicular-prostatic axis of prolactin synthesis and release from the pituitary, in males of all ages, warrants more intensive study. The heterogeneity of prolactin in serum may also vary with age and disease, and it is probable that not all immunoreactive prolactin is biologically active. Estradiol-17β certainly promotes prolactin release[163] although testosterone has little, if any, effect on pituitary prolactin content. Early bioassay studies of Asano[149] suggested that pituitary prolactin content increased after prostatectomy. The possible feedback control of the 5α-androstanediols on prolactin output has been mentioned earlier in this chapter.

There is a considerable body of evidence which would indicate that prolactin directly governs certain aspects of prostatic biochemistry, and some of the reports relating to this have been previously discussed. It would seem that prolactin can accentuate the effects of androgens in stimulating prostatic growth and function, and it is interesting that the presence of specific binding sites for the hormone on prostatic membranes has recently been demonstrated.[210,222] The steroid-prolactin interrelationship that influences the putative effect of prolactin on prostatic tissue requires consideration. Friesen and colleagues have described prolactin receptors with high specificity and affinity in female rat liver.[223] Estrogen treatment induced the receptor in male rat liver, but not after hypophysectomy. Removal of the pituitary in the female rat resulted in the loss of the prolactin receptor, and it was suggested, therefore, that plasma prolactin concentration probably regulates the prolactin receptor level.[224,255] Similar mechanisms are reported to control prolactin binding sites of the rat prostate,[226] except that estrogens inhibit the specific binding of ^{125}I-ovine prolactin to the membrane preparation. Furthermore, active protein synthesis was found necessary for the maintenance of the receptors,[226] and, obviously, with such a rapid turnover, regulation of their concentration would play a major role in controlling prolactin action and might well be influenced by aging.

At present, prolactin cannot be said to have a trophic effect on the prostate and it is difficult to ascribe a functional role for the prolactin receptor. Although Asano et al.[227] showed that administration of antiserum to prolactin decreased the weight of the prostate gland of the rabbit, our own studies[165] indicated that CB154 administration to male rats for 30 days failed to affect prostatic weight. Moreover, equivocal data were obtained on the effect of prolactin on adenyl cyclase, the activity of which was stimulated only in certain of the homogenates prepared from the different lobes. At the same time, in these studies prolactin did not appear to markedly influence androgen metabolism by the rat prostate, although other experiments (Table 10) and work from other groups provided evidence to the contrary.[228,229] It may be, however, that since experimental evidence indicates that prolactin tends to act synergistically with other hormones,[112,148,211,230] it is possible that the inconsistent effects caused by prolactin[165] could mean that the ideal system in vitro had not been realized.

Our ultrastructural studies with related electron microscope microanalysis, using EMMA-4 (Associated Electrical Industries, Manchester), did, however, indicate changes in the lateral lobe after CB154 treatment,[165] with a marked decrease in the zinc concentrations in most regions of the cell. Aragona and Friesen have subsequently reported[226] that prolactin receptors are localized in the dorsolateral lobes of the rat prostate.

C. A Direct Control of the Prostate

Currently available evidence indicated that the determination of circulating, plasma hormone concentrations has, as yet, failed to clearly define any real abnormality in the endocrine status of an individual that can be readily seen to be implicated in the etiology of prostatic disease. In our own research program, consideration was given to alternative routes which might allow for a testicular influence on the prostate and, thereby, explain the age-related changes that occur. Attention was directed to the anatomical link between the testis and prostate by the excurrent duct system, the seminiferous tubules, rete testis, vasa efferentia, epididymal ducts, and the vasa deferentia, which could provide a connection by which androgens reach the target organs without entering the general circulation. Skinner and Rowson[231,232] have shown previously that severing the vasa deferentia caused a reduction in weight and in the fructose and citric acid content of the ampullae, which could be restored by the infusion of testosterone along the vasa.

Preliminary studies were established[233] to test the hypothesis that a direct hormonal influence could similarly be imposed on the prostate. The results indicated that vasoligation reduced the activity of the DNA dependent-RNA polymerase in the ventral lobes of the rat prostate. Furthermore, [³H]testosterone, infused along the vasa, was preferentially taken up by the prostate and seminal vesicles, implying, therefore, the feasibility of normal passage of androgen from the testis via the vas deferentia.

Unilateral castration of the fetus[234,235] restricts the development of the ipsilateral genital structures, suggesting that testicular secretion is not distributed to the general circulation, but produces a local effect via the genital tract.

TABLE 10

Effect of Prolactin on C$_{19}$-Steroid Metabolism by Human Prostatic Tissue[a]

Precursor steroid	Hormone added (5 I.U.)	Tissue protein in cultured tissue (mg)	Specific Radioactivity (dpm/nmol/mg protein)					Total 5α-reduced steroids formed	Total 5α-reduced steroid/precursor steroid
			T	A	5αDHT	5αA	An		
Androstenedione	Control	1.45	—	84.9	47.0	428.7	238.7	714.4	5.8
	Ovine prolactin	1.86	—	99.5	41.2	299.5	165.1	505.8	2.7
Testosterone	Control	1.73	203.1	12.4	163.6	107.4	69.1	340.1	1.67
	Ovine prolactin	1.67	265.4	6.5	111.1	45.6	30.2	186.9	0.70

Note: T = testosterone; A = androstenedione; 5α-DHT = 5α-dihydrotestosterone; 5αA = 5α-androstane-3,17-dione and An = androsterone

[a]   Mean specific radioactivity of steroids isolated from human prostatic explants (benign prostatic hyperplasia) cultured with either [7α-³H]testosterone or [1,2-³H]androstenedione in the presence of ovine prolactin. Steroids were characterized after routine isotope dilution procedures.

From Harper, M. E., Pike, A., Peeling, W. B., and Griffiths, K., *J. Endocrinol.*, 60, 117, 1974. With permission.

Further studies of Pierrepoint et al.[236] provided added support for the hypothesis that the epididymis exercises a direct and unilateral androgenic control over the prostate. It was shown that unilateral castration and vasectomy reduced the activity of the DNA-dependent RNA polymerase of the ipsilateral lobes of the prostate. This was not observed after unilateral orchidectomy when the epididymis was not removed. Also the epididimides, in the absence of the testis, but maintained by exogenous testosterone, sustained the prostate gland at a level not achieved in their absence. Furthermore, the epididymis in the absence of ipsilateral gonad, but maintained by the contralateral testis, provided a greater sustaining influence on the prostate than did the testis and epididymis separated from the target organs by vasoligation.

The evidence, therefore, suggests that the epididymides modulate prostatic activity through an intact vas deferens. Subsequently,[237] it was shown that the concentrations of testosterone in the deferential and testicular veins of the dog were comparable and higher than in peripheral blood, further suggesting that the deferential vein serves as a direct transporting system for androgens from the epididymis to the prostatic complex. The venous drainage of the cauda epididymidis is solely through the deferential vein, which is generally severed at vasectomy. Ligation of this vein reduces the DNA and RNA content of the ventral lobe of the prostate and also the RNA polymerase activity. Fluorescent and radio-opaque material can be transferred from the deferential vein directly to the prostate,[238,239] and a study of the venous drainage of the canine prostate[240] supported the concept that a small retrograde flow of blood would take androgen-rich blood from the deferential vein into the prostate gland.

Therefore, man and dog, virtually alone in the animal kingdom in their susceptibility to prostatic hypertrophy, are species in which the vasa deferentia pass through the prostate to reach the urethra (Figure 10). This direct-control mechanism of the prostate should receive further investigation with regard to its possible role in inducing prostatic dysfunction, perhaps by a retrospective study of the incidence and type of prostatic dysfunction in men who have had vasectomies earlier in life.

V. PROLACTIN, THE ADRENAL GLAND, AND THE PROSTATE

There are a number of reports indicating a relationship between the adrenal gland and the prostate,[152,241-244] and it would seem that adrenocortical steroids, progesterone, and the adrenal androgens may all influence prostatic growth and function. Tisell[242] noted that cortisone induced growth and secretory activity of prostatic epithelium, an effect accentuated by estradiol-17β. Adrenal hyperplasia and urinary retention was observed[241] in mice with estrogen-induced prostatic hyperplasia. Subsequent adrenalectomy induced urinary flow; the prostate then appeared histologically normal; and elevated adrenal activity, resulting from estrogen-promoted release of ACTH, was considered a potential factor in the pathogenesis of, at least, prostatic hyperplasia. Certainly, estrogen-promoted ACTH release results in adrenal hyperplasia,[203,245] and estrogens increased the adrenal responsiveness to ACTH.[246] Progesterone administration also stimulated the growth of the ventral prostate of castrated rats and prevented involution of the gland in castrated, hypophysectomized, adrenalectomized animals.[247]

Although at present, there is little evidence that the adrenal gland is related in any way to prostatic disease, experiments of Farnsworth and from our laboratories[80,248] indicated that the adrenal C_{19}-steroids, DHA sulfate, DHA, and androstenedione were metabolized in vivo and in vitro by benign hypertrophic tissue (Table 4). DHA sulfate, a major secretory product of the human adrenal cortex and present in large quantities in plasma, offers a potentially large source of precursor for androgenic hormone formation by the prostate.

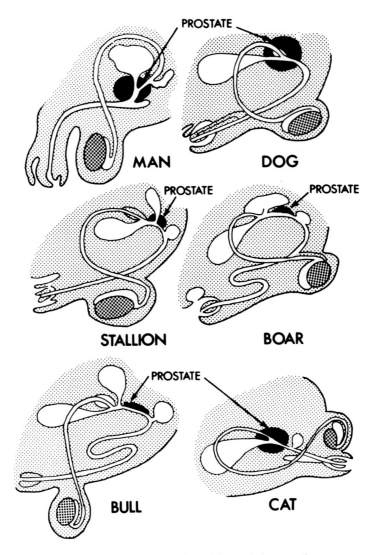

FIGURE 10.   Schematic representation of the genital tracts of various animals to illustrate the passage of the ductus deferens through the prostate of man and dog compared with those of the other domestic animals.

The influence of these adrenal C_{19}-steroids on prostatic tissue may be more significant, however, in patients with prostatic cancer treated by castration or estrogen therapy. Normally, administration of ACTH suppresses plasma testosterone levels in men,[249,250] and investigations of our own group.[251] on untreated patients with prostatic cancer showed that Synacthen® administration produced a similar suppression. Androstenedione levels in plasma increased after Synacthen® treatment. A similar Synacthen® test, undertaken after at least 6 months of estrogen therapy when plasma testosterone concentrations had been markedly decreased to below 70 ng/100 mℓ, resulted in an elevation in the concentrations of both androstenedione and testosterone, the latter showing a two- to ninefold increase. Plasma androstenedione levels in untreated patients did not differ significantly from those in elderly, control, hospitalized men (10 to 125 ng/100 mℓ), neither were they elevated after prolonged estrogen therapy. The plasma testosterone response to Synacthen® during the estrogen treatment may have been a result of increased DHA sulfate or DHA secretion, followed by peripheral conversion to testosterone. There is evidence, however, of a small direct secretion of testosterone by the adrenal gland,[72] and the adrenal synthesis of testosterone and its stimulation by Synacthen® has been demonstrated by human adrenal explants in organ culture.[252] These and other studies from the Institute[253] provided some of the first evidence that prolactin may influence the synthesis of C_{19}-steroids from the adrenal gland, and recent investigations of Vermeulen et al.[254] revealed that three males with prolactinomas and patients on psychotropic drugs with elevated plasma prolactin levels had significantly raised plasma concentrations of DHA and its sulfate. Furthermore, the findings of an increased urinary DHA excretion in patients with hyperprolactinemic amenorrhea[255] and hyperprolactinemia associated with bilateral adrenal hyperplasia[256] suggest a trophic effect of prolactin on the human adrenal gland. Specific binding sites for prolactin have also been reported in adrenal tissue,[223,257] and, in male rats and mice, ectopic pituitary isografts produced a significant elevation of prolactin levels with concomitant adrenal stimulation.[258] The relationship between DHA levels in the plasma with increasing age has been investigated by De Peretti and Forest,[259] and the changes in DHA concentration at early puberty associated with a possible "adrenarche" were discussed. Prolactin also must be considered a factor influencing sexual maturation during prepuberty and puberty.

It would seem, therefore, that the adrenal cortex of the patient receiving endocrine therapy for carcinoma of the prostate is responsive to ACTH, supporting earlier observations[260,261] that a secondary rise in plasma androgen concentration during therapy in some of these patients may be of adrenal origin. Dexamethasone treatment decreased plasma testosterone from 50 to 100 ng/100 mℓ to below the limits of detection.[141,262,263] Whether this secondary rise in plasma testosterone relates to a resumption of tumor growth, dissemination of the disease, and subsequent relapse is at present under study, but initial observations would indicate that it may not be the endocrine parameters but factors such as polyamines, carcinoembryonic antigen, α-fetoprotein, or other tumor markers that will provide the means of assessing recurrence and metastatic spread.

VI. ANDROGEN ACTION, HORMONE RECEPTORS, AND THE PROSTATE

A considerable weight of evidence supports the assumption that benign and malignant prostatic growth is androgen mediated. Plasma hormones may well have a permissive role in influencing this abnormal growth of prostatic tissue, but it would seem reasonable that attention should be directed to abnormalities within the target tissue itself. Indeed, there has been an underlying, fundamental assumption in many laboratories over the past decade that information on the endocrine disturbance inherent in prostatic disease will accrue from precise biochemical investigations into the cellular processes by which androgens control the growth and function of the gland. Such investigations, particularly with the ventral lobes of the rat prostate, clearly indicate that in the prostate, as in other steroid-responsive cells of other target tissues, steroid hormones function through a well-defined, integrated series of intracellular events, the most important of which is probably the association of the steroid with a cytoplasmic "receptor" protein, through which the hormone elicits the initial transcriptional processes at specific nuclear "receptor" sites.[113] The selective binding of a particular steroid, followed by translocation to the nucleus and the specific binding of the steroid-receptor complex to these nuclear acceptor sites, thereby regulates gene expression, as

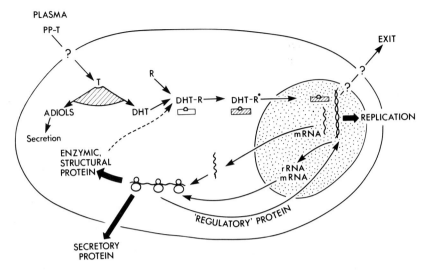

FIGURE 11.   Schematic representation of the effects of androgens within the prostatic cell, depicting the essential characteristics of the mechanism of steroid action. T, testosterone; DHT, 5α-dihydrotestosterone; Adiols, the various androstanediols; PP, plasma proteins responsible for the transport of testosterone (SHBG in man); R, specific intracellular receptor; DHT-R, steroid-receptor complex; DHT-R*, the active complex; mRNA and rRNA, messenger and ribosomal ribonucleic acid respectively. Question marks refer to processes not completely elucidated; thick arrows relate to processes of growth and function, dotted arrows to theoretical relationships, and thin arrows to the development of processes within the cell.

illustrated in Figure 11. It is interesting that, with other target tissues, circulating hormones such as estradiol-17β or aldosterone bind to receptor and are then translocated to the nucleus, whereas in the prostate, testosterone is converted to the "intracellular hormone", 5α-dihydrotestosterone, before translocation to the nucleus. Detailed information on the mechanism of action of androgens has recently been discussed,[264] but essentially the steroid-receptor complex regulates transcription, gene activation, and the integrated processes related to growth.

The precise mechanism by which testosterone enters the prostatic cell is, as yet, poorly defined, but some degree of selectivity is probably involved,[265] and plasma SHBG will influence steroid entry. Current evidence suggests that the nonprotein-bound testosterone crosses the plasma membrane and is metabolized to a variety of 5α-reduced steroids (Figure 3), although high levels of SHBG have been found associated with the stroma of the hypertrophied prostate.[266,267] As stated earlier, 5α-androstanediols and unmetabolized testosterone may have roles in physiological processes independent of receptor or transcription, but 5α-dihydrotestosterone is retained by the receptor proteins of selective high affinity; the steroid-receptor complex then attains a conformation with increased affinity for nuclear components and is then translocated to the chromatin where it is retained to initiate and promote the cellular mechanisms leading to tissue growth. After some time, the 5α-dihydrotestosterone leaves the nucleus by some, as yet, ill-defined mechanism and may well be secreted directly from the prostate or further metabolized. In effect, therefore, the process is concerned in maintaining an effective intracellular concentration of active 5α-dihydrotestosterone-receptor complex to control normal prostatic function.

It is reasonable, therefore, that since prostatic dysfunction may originate from an age-dependent imbalance of C_{19}-steroid metabolism, resulting in localized androgenic stimulation, the intracellular formation of 5α-dihydrotestosterone has received considerable attention. The reported age-dependent accumulation of this steroid in the prostate gland of elderly men without concomitant change in testosterone concentration, particularly in the periurethral area,[167] may result in localized stimulation. Enzymatic imbalance, facilitated steroid entry, or inhibited release of androgen may, therefore, result in prostatic dysfunction. Of interest in relation to the high concentration of 5α-dihydrotestosterone in hypertrophy are the reports of a lower conversion of testosterone to 5α-dihydrotestosterone in neoplastic tissue.[268,269] Since testosterone also binds to the androgen-receptor protein,[270] the resultant testosterone-receptor complex may well elicit cellular responses which, in the absence of the normal 5α-dihydrotestosterone regulation, could induce prostatic dysfunction. A higher conversion of 5α-dihydrotestosterone to 5α-androstane-3α,17β-diol has recently been implicated in prostatic hypertrophy[271] with the diol exerting some effect on cell growth in a situation corresponding to the canine prostate, but in other studies[171,272] this conversion has been reported to be minimal. Moreover, the evidence would indicate that 5α-androstane-3α,17β-diol usually exerts its action through conversion to 5α-dihydrotestosterone[273] and normally does not bind significantly to the androgen receptor.[274] Furthermore, although it can eventually induce benign growth of the prostate of castrated dogs,[133] it may not be the active androgen or androstanediol of this tissue.[96,275] Extranuclear, receptor-independent effects of the androstanediols on other sites in the cell cannot be excluded from a consideration of etiology. Therefore, although an imbalance in the C_{19}-steroid metabolic pattern of the prostate cell may be functionally concerned in promoting benign or malignant growth, the presentation of an increased concentration of intracellular androgen might be dependent on an elevated level of effective receptor protein. Formation of the steroid-receptor complex is a prerequisite for steroid hormone action, and abnormal prostatic growth may result from an overloading of the receptor-acceptor-gene system with consequent lack of control of the regulatory unit (Figure 11).

A. Receptors in Human Prostatic Tissue

Considerable effort has been directed to the characterization and quantitation of steroid-binding components of the human prostate. This work has recently been the subject of a review by Davies,[276] who considered the clinical possibilities and limitations of receptor analysis in relation to its inherent, technological difficulties, one of the principal being tissue contamination with SHBG, considered by some[266] a potential reservoir of androgen within prostatic cells. Also discussed[276] was the procedure used in the Tenovus Institute for the measurement in human tissue of total receptor site concentration in which receptor is first stabilized by protamine sulfate precipitation.[277,278]

Figure 12 illustrates results that have been obtained from our own studies with sucrose density gradient centrifugation, Figures 12a, b, and c showing that labeling of cytosol preparations from normal, carcinomatous, and hypertrophic prostate, respectively, with [³H]5α-dihydrotestosterone yields two peaks of radioactivity with sedimentation coefficients in the ranges 3 to 4S and 7 to 8S. Evidence for the specificity and low capacity of the 7 to 8S peak, the cytoplasmic receptor, has been previously described.[279,280] 5α-Dihydrotestosterone localization within the nucleus[281] due to translocation of the cytoplasmic steroid-receptor complex has been reported,[279,280] together with the marked stimulation by the complex of chromatin transcription by RNA polymerase.[279,282,283] Figure 12d shows a sedimentation profile of [³H]5α-dihydrotestosterone-receptor complex derived from salt extraction of a hypertrophied prostate nuclear preparation previously incubated with prelabeled cytosol. The characteristic single peak of protein-bound radioactivity corresponds to the nuclear 5α-dihydrotestosterone-receptor complex with sedimentation coefficient of approximately 4S.

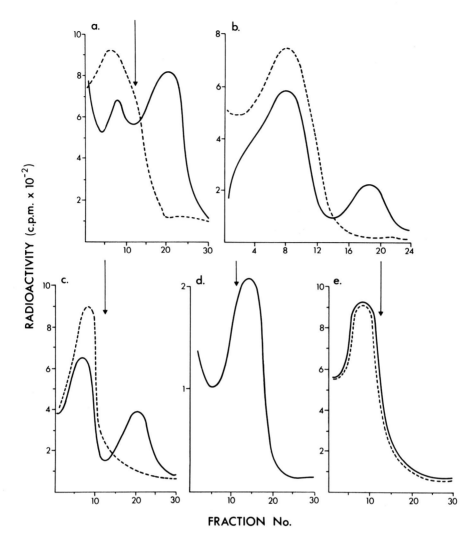

FIGURE 12.   Sedimentation analysis of [³H]5α-dihydrotestosterone binding components in human prostate subcellular fractions. Samples of normal, hypertrophied or neoplastic prostate were homogenized and subcellular fractions prepared as previously described.[279] Aliquots of cytosols (100,000 × g supernatant) were incubated (1 hr at 0 to 4°C) with [³H]DHT (4 nmol/ℓ) in the absence (   ) and presence of (- - -) of unlabeled DHT (400 nmol/ℓ). Portions (400 $\mu\ell$) of ³H-labeled cytosols were layered on linear 5 mℓ sucrose gradients (5 to 20% w/v) and centrifuged at 100,000 × g_{av} for 16 hr at 0 to 4°C in a Beckman L2-65B or L5-65B ultracentrifuge using a SW50.1 (6 × 5 mℓ) swinging bucket rotor (r_{av} 8.35 cm). Gradients were fractionated by upward displacement with 40 to 50% (w/v) sucrose and approximately 30 fractions were collected in scintillation vials. Attempts were made to label nuclear receptors by the incubation of ³H-labeled cytosol with equal volumes of prostate nuclei for 15 min at 37°C. Nuclei were sedimented, washed several times with buffer to remove free [³H]steroid and extranuclear [³H]steroid-receptor complex, and then extracted with KCl (0.4 mol/ℓ). Nuclear debris was sedimented from the viscous extract by centrifugation at 100,000 g_{av} for 10 to 30 min and samples of salt-extract examined on sucrose gradients containing an uniform concentration of KCl (0.5 mol/ℓ) as described for cytosol. Profiles obtained from such studies on cytosol from human normal prostate (a), human hypertrophied prostate (b), and human neoplastic prostate (c), and on nuclei from human hypertrophied prostate (d). Also shown is an example of human hypertrophied prostate exhibiting no low-capacity binding components (e). Throughout, the direction of centrifugation was from left to right and the sedimentation marker (arrow) was bovine serum albumin ($S_{20,w}$ 4.6S).

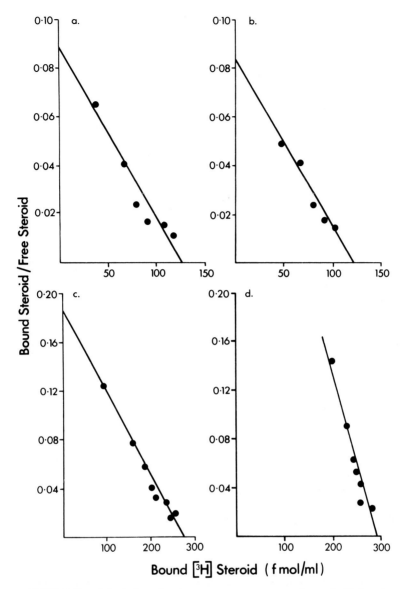

FIGURE 13.   Calculation of androgen-receptor concentration and affinity of androgen-receptor interaction. Values for specific androgen binding were subjected to
Scatchard-type analysis so that the concentration of receptor ([R]) and the dissociation constants for androgen-receptor interaction (K_D) could be calculated. Representative results are shown in this figure. (a) Androgen receptor from human normal
prostate cytosol: [R] = 52 fmol/mg protein, K_D = 1.6 nmol/ℓ. (b) Androgen receptor from human hypertrophied prostate cytosol: [R] = 56.6 fmol/mg protein, K_D
= 1.48 nmol/ℓ. (d) Androgen receptor from human prostate cancer cytosol: [R]
= 63 fmol/mg protein, K_D = 0.69 nmol/ℓ.

B. Levels of Androgen Receptors in Human Prostatic Tissue

The determination in our laboratories of androgen receptor proteins in normal, hypertrophic, and carcinomatous prostate tissue by saturation analysis, using the protamine sulfate procedure, indicated in all cases the presence of one class of high-affinity
binding sites (Figure 13). Specific [³H]5α-dihydrotestosterone-binding components
were present in nuclear and cytoplasmic preparations of all samples of prostatic tissue

TABLE 11

Androgen Receptors in Human Prostate Subcellular Fractions

Fraction	Tissue		Receptor concentration		Cytoplasmic Nuclear	Dissociation constant (nmol/1)
			fmol	Molecules/cell		
Cytosol	Normal	Central	44—52	1218—1231	1.514	0.99—1.60
		Peripheral	53—57	1041—1354	1.33	1.01—1.29
	Hypertrophy		38—92	2423—5461	1.49	1.56—2.81
	Cancer		63	3363	2.20	0.69
Nuclei	Normal	Central	196—223	758—860		1.33—4.99
		Peripheral	221—248	850—955		1.03—1.30
	Hypertrophy		412—868	1387—3922		1.17—1.41
	Cancer		546	1529		0.39

Note: Concentrations of cytoplasmic receptor are expressed as fmol/mg protein and those of nuclear receptor as fmol/mg DNA. Values shown are the range of concentrations obtained in this series of experiments.

analyzed, and values for receptor-site concentration for occupied plus unoccupied sites, obtained by incubation at 15°C for 16 hr, are given in Table 11.[276] The unoccupied sites contributed between 2 and 30% of the total, but were usually less than 10%, in line with a previous report.[284]

The amount of data is limited, but assessment of the results available does suggest a higher cellular content of androgen receptors in hypertrophic and malignant prostatic tissue, with a less efficient translocation process in the neoplastic state implicated by the cytoplasmic receptor to nuclear receptor ratio. Furthermore, the apparent dissociation constants imply a higher affinity of ligand-receptor interaction in the malignant tissue. It will be important to determine whether there are different receptor characteristics in the various cells and areas of the prostate which might relate to the occurrence of hypertrophy or carcinoma, since molecular rearrangement may affect affinity for 5α-dihydrotestosterone, for another metabolite of testosterone or possibly for estradiol-17β. Further data will accumulate, and it will be most interesting to find whether these preliminary differences are maintained.

It has always been hoped that the analysis of androgen receptors in carcinoma of the prostate may be valuable in determining the potential value of endocrine therapy for the treatment of the disease in a manner simiar to the situation found in studies of breast cancer. Estradiol-17β receptor analysis of breast tumor tissue has been found of value in predicting the response to hormone therapy.[285] Since certain chemotherapeutic agents are considered to act through an interaction with the receptor,[286,287] then the presence of the receptor protein would be indicative of the potential effect of such antiandrogens in inducing tumor response. Treatment of prostatic cancer is, however, the subject of another chapter of this volume. It is noteworthy at this stage, however, to emphasize the relatively unpleasant side effects of diethylstilbestrol generally used in the treatment of prostatic carcinoma. Cardiovascular problems, gynecomastia, and loss of libido are relatively common, and, yet, the steroidal compounds with supposed antiandrogenic properties are comparatively ineffective.[287] It must be hoped that the extensive knowledge gained during the past decade into the mechanism by which androgenic hormones regulate prostatic function may eventually be of value in the development of a more effective therapy, possibly with nonsteroidal compounds such as flutamide.[288-290]

C. Other Receptor Proteins in Prostatic Tissue

Over the past few years evidence has been found for the presence in prostatic tissue of specific estrogen receptors.[291-293] High affinity binding in the absence of 5α-dihydrotestosterone binding was reported in benign prostatic adenomas,[292] whereas Wagner and colleagues[291] found receptors for both 5α-dihydrotestosterone and estradiol-17β in normal and hypertrophic tissue. None of the prostatic tissue in our laboratory investigations was found to have estradiol-17β receptors when studied with standard dextran-charcoal adsorption techniques and competition with unlabeled diethylstilbestrol. Endogenous estrogen was not replaced, however. It has already been stated earlier in this chapter that a more direct role has often been assumed for estradiol-17β in the pathogenesis of prostatic dysfunction, and the presence of these estradiol-17β receptor proteins tends to suggest the presence of an estrogen regulatory mechanism in the prostatic cell, although its physiological significance must await further investigation. It may well be that such a process functions merely to remove estrogens from the androgen dominated cellular processes.

Furthermore, an investigation to determine whether the estradiol-17β receptor is localized in stromal or epithelial tissue should be interesting, since stromal and epithelial tissues respond differently to hormones[294] and may well have a different receptor status. Progesterone receptorlike binding in stromal tissue, rather than epithelial tissue, has already been described by Cowan et al.[295] Although stromal tissue possesses a 5α-reductase, metabolizes C_{19}-steroids[80] and responds in organ culture to androgens,[296] the presence of estradiol-17β and progesterone receptors certainly suggests a different hormonal control mechanism, further elucidation of which may be of interest in relation to prostatic disease. Recent unpublished preliminary studies of Pierrepoint and Chaisiri[338] have indicated that most of the estrogen receptor of the dog prostate appears to be located in the stromal tissue.

VII. ENVIRONMENTAL ASPECTS OF PROSTATIC CARCINOMA

In the foregoing discussions attention was drawn to McNeal's hypothesis[19,22] that prostatic carcinoma originates in active epithelial tissue rather than from regions of atrophy. The hypothesis does not, however, assign the role of prostatic carcinogen to the androgens. Indeed, the evidence tends to indicate that the androgenic hormones have more of a permissive role than one of induction in the promotion of prostatic neoplasia. A change in the general hormonal status or an increased sensitivity to either androgen or estrogen may predispose the prostate gland to respond to some exogenous stimulus. Lasnitzki,[297] for example, demonstrated that estrogens enhanced the hyperplastic effect resulting from the incubation of rat prostatic explants with the carcinogen methylcholanthrene.

There is now some evidence that viruses are, at least, associated with human tumors and there are many who now argue strongly for an association of RNA oncogenic viruses with prostatic cancer. Ultrastructural studies have identified viruslike particles in prostatic carcinoma,[298-300] and there is convincing evidence for an etiological role for viruses in certain other animal malignancies.[301] The possibility, therefore, that a viral agent may be implicated in prostatic carcinoma in man should be borne in mind, although a recent epidemiological study[302] indicated that there was no evidence to support any relationship between a venereally transmissible oncogenic agent and the disease, despite the suggested association between prostatic cancer and excessive sexual activity.[32]

Rotkin's report,[302] however, directed attention to the possible risk to man from an environmental or industrial source, and it is interesting in this respect, that a number of investigations have described an increased mortality from prostatic cancer among workers exposed to the heavy metal cadmium.[303-306] It was suggested[307] that replacement of intracellular prostatic zinc with cadmium may affect cellular function and promote neoplasia. The clinical effects of cadmium on the male reproductive tract are well established,[308,309] and it is known[308] that parenteral administration of zinc prior to cadmium to experimental animals prevents testicular damage. These, and other studies, over the past 20 years[310-312] have been concerned with understanding the mechanism by which cadmium affects the testis, and evidence suggested that its primary target was the vascular supply of this gland.[313] The relationship between zinc and cadmium in the reproductive system of the rat was investigated by Gunn et al.,[314] who also concluded that the principal effect of cadmium was on the testes and the subsequent decrease in plasma androgen levels resulted in a marked fall in prostatic weight. Testicular synthesis of testosterone in vitro was impaired after cadmium administration,[315] and subsequent studies[316,317] suggested that there was no direct effect of cadmium on the prostate gland.

The implication that cadmium could be a potential carcinogen in animals and man[303,305,306,317] stimulated, in our laboratories, an interest in the effect of the metal on the lateral prostate of the rat,[318,319] which is known to contain high concentrations of zinc.[320] Its uptake is influenced by various hormones[321,322] and is also affected by cadmium.[310] Although cadmium administration in vivo resulted in a decreased plasma concentration of testosterone and an elevated level of LH, ultrastructural studies[319] clearly suggested that cadmium exerts a direct effect on the lateral lobe of the prostate. Electron microscope microanalysis using EMMA-4 indicated that there were large reductions in the levels of zinc in all subcellular regions of the epithelial cells of the lateral lobe soon after cadmium administration. Cadmium was found localized in the nucleoli and lysosomes of the epithelium. An interesting feature of the study was the reaction of the basal cells which appeared not to be adversely affected by the presence of cadmium. On the contrary, apparent stimulation of these cells was observed, and there was an increased pinocytotic activity at the basement membrane. There were no involutionary changes as was seen in the epithelial cell, and it is interesting that, in a separate investigation,[323] basal cells also responded differently to hormonal changes, being seen to proliferate after castration. Incubation of cadmium in vitro with explants of lateral prostate of rat[318] produced similar results, with the metal entering the cell, causing local necrosis and subsequent proliferation of basal cells. Basal cell growth also has been observed after administration of 20-methylcholanthrene directly into the prostate,[324] and it would seem that their potential for rapid growth is in relation to a hormonal or physiological environment which does not promote the normal function and maintenance of the prostatic epithelial cell.

These observations serve to emphasize that the various cell types of the prostate gland, the epithelial cells, muscle fibers, basal cells, fibroblasts, etc. do not respond in a similar manner to changes in the hormonal environment. The basis of the major advances in recent years in our understanding of the mechanism of hormone action at the molecular level has been primarily centered on the epithelial cell as the principal target. There have been comparatively few biochemical studies which were directly concerned with the interrelationship between the epithelial and stromal elements of the prostate gland. It is noteworthy, however, that in benign prostatic hypertrophy the normal, coordinated growth pattern of the epithelial and stromal cells in the periurethral tissue is disturbed to produce adenomata, which are not of one-cell type, but contain varying proportions of the various cellular components,[325] although one particular cell type may well predominate. The extent to which hormones control the growth and development of the stromal elements is at present not very clear, and more fundamental work is required on the coordinated growth processes that would seem to control the interrelationship between epithelial and stromal elements in the prostate gland.[294] Equally important are more definitive studies of the cells of the various zones of the prostate gland, investigations which may provide more insight into the reasons why the epithelial tissue of the peripheral zone of the human prostate is predominantly the site of origin of carcinoma. Moreover, the differences between this type of androgen-dependent, prostatic, epithelial cell and those of other male, sex-accessory glands which rarely develop cancer remain to be elucidated. Any changes in circulating hormones with increasing age must affect these other glands of the male urogenital system, and, again, intensive studies into the effects of aging on fundamental biochemical processes within these various cell types would seem warranted.

There is evidence from cell culture[326] that elevated intracellular levels of cAMP may be concerned in contact inhibition, whereby cultured cells cease dividing when contact is made with other cells. Goldberg et al.[327] have also implicated cGMP in these control mechanisms and suggest that concentrations of these two cyclic nucleotides are inversely related in regulating biochemical processes concerned with cell growth. The effect of various protein hormones, prolactin, GH, FSH, etc. which normally act through membrane-receptors, with consequent stimulation of adenyl cyclase and elevation of cAMP concentrations, on such a regulatory system within the various cells of the prostate could well be interesting.

Other aspects of prostatic intracellular biochemistry should also be considered in relation to neoplasia. The high concentration of aliphatic polyamines in prostatic tissue and in seminal fluid has been well documented.[328-330] Although one of these studies[330] clearly demonstrated a relationship between the levels of spermine in seminal plasma and sperm count and motility, the role of the polyamines in human reproduction is still uncertain.[329] It is well established, however, that polyamines can influence intracellular macromolecular synthesis in prostatic preparations.[328,331] They have a marked effect on RNA transcription and translocation stabilization of the membranes of the endoplasmic reticulum; they interact with polyribosomes and inhibit nucleolytic enzymes.[328,331-333] The reported increase in the spermidine to spermine ratio in rapidly proliferating neoplastic tissue and associated elevation in the activity of ornithine-decarboxylase, an enzyme concerned in polyamine biosynthesis,[334] also directs attention to the relationship between polyamines and DNA replication. Whether the use of specific and sensitive analysis for the measurement of polyamine levels in plasma and seminal fluid will reflect abnormal growth patterns within prostatic tissue remains to be determined, but recent investigations by Russell[335,336] offer considerable encouragement. Also important in relation to etiology is the suggestion of Williams-Ashman et al.[328] that the oxidation of spermine or spermidine by certain amine oxidases present in seminal plasma and, possibly, in microbial enzymes present in the prostate to aldehydic oxidation products may be deleterious to the prostatic cells. Such oxidation products are cytotoxic and their potential carcinogenic effect requires further consideration.

It was stated at the beginning of this review that prostatic disease, benign hyperplasia or malignant neoplasia, represents a major clinical problem affecting a large proportion of elderly men. Of all species, it appears that only the aging dog is similarly afflicted. Whether this species susceptibility is a function of changes in the pattern of circulating hormones with age and/or alterations in the sensitivity and interaction of the various cellular elements of the prostate in association with environmental factors shared by these two animals remains to be determined.

It has long been accepted in man that, after the early period of prostatic growth during adolescence, the size of the gland remains relatively stable until the fifth decade when hypertrophy and sometimes carcinoma can then be found. Prostatic disease is related to the aging process. Relevant, however, are the studies of MacMahon et al.[337] which drew attention to the decreased risk from breast cancer in women who had an early pregnancy, suggesting hormonal changes in the breast tissue during this adolescent period of life may "trigger" certain biochemical events, which, later in life, become manifest as neoplastic growth or, conversely, protects against it. Endocrinologists will no doubt be directing their attention to this early phase in the life of women in an attempt to understand these "risk or protective factors" and equally, in the male, prostatic disease may result in the elderly man as a consequence of endocrine changes established in the adolescent youth. In this respect, the recent report from Rotkin[302] is most interesting. A detailed study of patients with prostatic cancer suggested that a delayed onset of sexuality in the late adolescent period with an early suppression of sexual activity were characteristics prevalent in those with the disease. A shorter span of sexual activity may then relate to prostatic cancer, with interest centering on the late pubertal phase of the male life as a period of cancer initiation, when the potential cancer patient may be endocrinologically different from the "normal" male. Whatever the outcome, however, the importance of the epidemiological approach to our understanding of the etiology of prostatic carcinoma is becoming steadily more evident.

VIII. ACKNOWLEDGMENTS

The authors gratefully acknowledge the financial support of the Tenovus organization. They are also indebted to Mrs. Margaret Lewis, the Institute Secretary, who typed and corrected the manuscript and Mr. Stephen McAllister, Head of the Medical Illustration Unit of the Institute, who prepared the figures.

REFERENCES

1. Hunter, J., *Observations on Certain Parts of the Animal Oeconomy,* 1st ed., Bibliotheca Osteriana, London, 1786, 39.
2. White, J. W., The results of double castration in hypertrophy of the prostate, *Ann. Surg.,* 22, 1, 1895.
3. Cabot, A. T., The question of castration for enlarged prostate, *Ann. Surg.,* 24, 265, 1896.
4. Huggins, C. and Clark, P. J., Quantitative studies of prostatic secretion. II. The effect of castration and of estrogen injection on the normal and on the hyperplastic prostatic glands of dogs, *J. Exp. Med.,* 72, 747, 1940.
5. Huggins, C. and Hodges, C. V., Studies on prostatic cancer. I. The effect of castration, of estrogen and of androgen injection on serum phosphatases in metastatic carcinoma of the prostate, *Cancer Res.,* 1, 293, 1941.
6. Huggins, C., Stevens, R. E., Jr., and Hodges, C. V., Studies on prostatic cancer. II. The effects of castration on advanced carcinoma of the prostate gland, *Arch. Surg. (Chicago),* 43, 209, 1941.
7. Ferguson, J. D., Castration and oestrogen therapy, in *Endocrinology of Malignant Disease,* Stoll, B. A., Ed., W. B. Saunders, London, 1972, 247.
8. Franks, L. M., Latent carcinoma of prostate, *J. Pathol. Bacteriol.,* 68, 603, 1954.
9. Franks, L. M., Benign nodular hyperplasia of the prostate. A review, *Ann. R. Coll. Surg. Engl.,* 14, 92, 1954.
10. Sommers, S. C., Endocrine changes with prostatic carcinoma, *Cancer (Philadelphia),* 10, 345, 1957.
11. Liavag, I., Atrophy and regenerationthe pathogenesis of prostatic carcinoma, *Acta Pathol. Microbiol. Scand.,* 73, 338, 1968.
12. Armenian, H. K., Lilienfeld, A. M., Diamond, E. L., and Bross, I. D. J., Relation between benign prostatic hypertrophy and cancer of the prostate. A prospective and retrospective study, *Lancet,* 115, 1974.
13. Vital statistics and causes of death, World Health Statistics Annual Report, Vol. 1, World Health Organization, Geneva, 1971.
14. Labess, M., Occult carcinoma in clinically benign hypertrophy of the prostate: a pathological and clinical study, *J. Urol.,* 68, 893, 1952.

15. **Turner, R. D. and Belt, E.,** The results of 1694 consecutive simple perineal prostatectomies, *J. Urol.*, 77, 853, 1957.

16. **Greenwald, P., Kirmss, V., Polan, A. K., and Dick, V. S.,** Cancer of the prostate among men with benign prostatic hyperplasia, *J. Natl. Cancer Inst.*, 53, 335, 1974.

17. **Rotkin, I. D.,** Epidemiology of benign prostatic hypertrophy: review and speculations, in *Benign Prostatic Hyperplasia,* Grayhack, J. T., Wilson, J. D., and Scherbenske, M. J., Eds., National Institutes of Health, Bethesda, Md., 1975, 105.

18. **Franks, L. M.,** Benign prostatic hyperplasia, *Lancet,* 2, 293, 1974.

19. **McNeal, J. E.,** Age related changes in prostatic epithelium associated with carcinoma, in *Some Aspects of the Aetiology and Biochemistry of Prostatic Cancer,* 3rd Tenovus Workshop, Griffiths, K. and Pierrepoint, C. G., Eds., Alpha Omega Alpha, Cardiff, 1970, 23.

20. **Franks, L. M.,** In *Some Aspects of the Aetiology and Biochemistry of Prostatic Cancer,* 3rd Tenovus Workshop, Griffiths, K. and Pierrepoint, C. G., Eds., Alpha Omega Alpha, Cardiff, 1970, 39.

21. **McNeal, J. E.,** The prostate and prostatic urethra, a morphologic synthesis, *J. Urol.,* 107, 1008, 1972.

22. **McNeal, J. E.,** Structure and pathology of the prostate, in *Normal and Abnormal Growth of the Prostate,* Goland, M., Ed., Charles C Thomas, Springfield, Ill., 1975, 55.

23. **Lowsley, O. S.,** The development of the human prostate gland with reference to the development of other structures at the neck of the urinary bladder, *Am. J. Anat.,* 13, 299, 1912.

24. **Blacklock, N. J.,** Surgical anatomy of the prostate, in *Scientific Foundation of Urology,* Vol. 2, Williams, D. I. and Chisholm, G. D., Eds., Year Book Medical Publishing, Chicago, 1976, 113.

25. **Koppel, M., Heranze, D. R., and Shimkin, M. B.,** Characteristics of patients with prostatic carcinoma: a control case study on 83 autopsy pairs, *J. Urol.,* 98, 229, 1967.

26. **Reischauer, F.,** Die entstehung der sogenannten prostate hypertrophie, *Virchows Arch. Pathol. Anat. Physiol.,* 256, 357, 1925.

27. **Varkarakis, M., Castro, J. E., and Azzopardi, J. G.,** Prognosis of stage 1 carcinoma of the prostate, *Proc. R. Soc. Med.,* 63, 91, 1970.

28. **Correa, R. J., Anderson, R. G., Gibbons, R. P., and Tate, M. J.,** Latent carcinoma of the prostate — why the controversy?, *J. Urol.,* 111, 644, 1974.

29. **Hirst, A. E., Jr. and Bergman, R. T.,** Carcinoma of the prostate in men 80 or more years old, *Cancer (Philadelphia),* 7, 136, 1954.

30. **Greenwald, P., Damon, A., Kirmss, V., and Polan, A. K.,** Physical and demographic features of men before developing cancer of the prostate, *J. Natl. Cancer Inst.,* 53, 341, 1974.

31. **King, H., Diamond, E., and Lilienfeld, A. M.,** Some epidemiological aspects of cancer of the prostate, *J. Chronic Dis.,* 16, 117, 1963.

32. **Steele, R., Lees, R. E. M., Kraus, A. S., and Rao, C.,** Sexual factors in the epidemiology of cancer of the prostate *J. Chronic. Dis.,* 24, 29, 1971.

33. **Kessler, H.,** Cancer mortality among diabetics, *J. Natl. Cancer Inst.,* 44, 673, 1970.

34. **Lea, A. J.,** Diabetes mellitus and neoplasia, *Lancet,* 1, 821, 1966.

35. **Bourke, J. B. and Griffin, J. P.,** Diabetes mellitus in patients with benign prostatic hyperplasia, *Br. Med. J.,* 4, 492, 1968.

36. **Wynder, E. L., Mabuchi, K., and Whitmore, W. F.,** Epidemiology of cancer of the prostate, *Cancer (Philadelphia),* 28, 344, 1971.

37. **Buell, P. and Dunn, J. E.,** Cancer mortality among Japanese Issei and Nissei of California, *Cancer (Philadelphia),* 18, 656, 1965.

38. **Haenszel, W. and Kurihara, M.,** Studies of Japanese migrants. I. Mortality from cancer and other diseases among Japanese in the United States, *J. Natl. Cancer Inst.,* 40, 43, 1968.

39. **Kobayashi, T., Labotsky, J., and Lloyd, C. W.,** Plasma testosterone and urinary 17-ketosteroids in Japanese and Occidentals, *J. Clin. Endocrinol. Metab.,* 26, 610, 1966.

40. **Ibayashi, H., Fujita, T., Motohashi, K., Yoshida, S., Ohsawa, N., Murakawa, S., Yokota, T., and Okinaka, S.,** Determination of adrenocorticotrophin in human urine by a benzoic-acid adsorption method, *J. Clin. Endocrinol. Metab.,* 21, 140, 1961.

41. **Okamoto, M., Setoishi, C., Horiuchi, Y., Mashimo, K., Moriji, K., and Itoh, S.,** Urinary excretion of testosterone and epitestosterone and plasma levels of LH and testosterone in the Japanese and Ainu, *J. Clin. Endocrinol. Metab.,* 32, 673, 1971.

42. **Kent, J. R. and Acone, A. B.,** Plasma testosterone levels and aging in males, in Androgens in Normal and Pathological Conditions, Vermeulen, A. and Exley, D., Eds., *Excerpta Med. Int. Congr. Ser.,* 101, 31, 1966.

43. **Vermeulen, A., Rubens, R., and Verdonck, L.,** Testosterone secretion and metabolism in male senescence, *J. Clin. Endocrinol.,* 34, 730, 1972.

44. **Pirke, K. M. and Doerr, P.,** Age related changes and interrelationship between plasma testosterone, oestradiol and testosterone-binding globulin in normal adult males, *Acta Endocrinol. (Copenhagen),* 74, 792, 1973.

45. **Mahoudeau, J. A., Delassalle, A., and Bricaire, H.,** Secretion of dihydrotestosterone by human prostate in benign prostatic hypertrophy, *Acta Endocrinol. (Copenhagen),* 77, 401, 1974.

46. **Frick, J.,** Danstellung einer methode zur bestimmung des testosteronspeigels in plasma und studie über den testosteronmetabolismus bein Mann über 60 Jahre, *Urol. Int.,* 24, 481, 1969.

47. **Nieschlag, E., Kley, K. H., Wiegelmann, W., Solbach, H. G., and Krüskemper, H. L.,** Lebensalter und endokrine funktion der testes des erwachsenen mannes, *Dtsch. Med. Wochenschr.,* 98, 1281, 1973.

48. **Kley, H. K., Nieschlag, E., Bidlingmaier, F., and Krüskemper, H. L.,** Possible age-dependent influence of estrogens on the binding of testosterone in plasma of adult men, *Horm. Metab. Res.,* 6, 213, 1974.

49. **Kelch, R. P., Jenner, M. R., Weinstein, R., Kaplan, S. L., and Grumbach, M. M.,** Estradiol and testosterone secretion by human, simian and canine testes, in males with hypogonadism and in male pseudohermaphrodites with feminising testes syndrome, *J. Clin. Invest.,* 51, 824, 1972.

50. **Longcope, C., Widrich, W., and Sawin, C. T.,** The secretion of estrone and estradiol-17β by human testis, *Steroids,* 20, 439, 1972.

51. **Weinstein, R., Kelch, R. P., Jenner, M. R., Kaplan, S. L., and Grumbach, M. M.,** Secretion of unconjugated androgens and estrogens by the normal and abnormal human testis before and after human chorionic gonadotrophin, *J. Clin. Invest.,* 53, 1, 1974.

52. **Longcope, C., Kato, T., and Horton, R.,** Conversion of blood androgens to estrogens in normal adult men and women, *J. Clin. Invest.,* 48, 2191, 1969.

53. **MacDonald, P. C., Grodin, J. M., and Siiteri, P. K.,** Dynamics of androgen and oestrogen secretion, in *Control of Gonadal Steroid Secretion,* Baird, D. T. and Strong, J. A., Eds., Williams & Wilkins, Baltimore, 1972, 157.

54. **Bardin, C. W. and Lipsett, M. B.,** Testosterone and androstenedione blood production rates in normal women and women with idiopathic hirsutism and polycystic ovaries, *J. Clin. Invest.,* 46, 891, 1967.

55. **Hemsell, D. L., Grodin, J. M., Brenner, P. F., Siiteri, P. K., and MacDonald, P. C.,** Plasma precursors of estrogen. II. Correlation of the extent of conversion of plasma androstenedione to estrogen with age, *J. Clin. Endocrinol.,* 38, 476, 1974.

56. **Kley, H. K., Nieschlag, E., and Krüskemper, H. L.,** Age dependence of plasma oestrogen response to HCG and ACTH in man, *Acta Endocrinol. (Copenhagen),* 79, 95, 1975.

57. **Doerr, P. and Pirke, K. M.,** Regulation of plasma oestrogens in normal adult males. I. Response of oestradiol, oestrone and testosterone to HCG and fluoxymesterone administration, *Acta Endocrinol. (Copenhagen),* 75, 617, 1974.

58. **Antoniades, N. H., Daughaday, W. H., and Slaunwhite, W. R.,** in *Hormones in Human Plasma,* Antoniades, N. H., Ed., Little, Brown, Boston, 1960, 455.

59. **Mercier, C. and Baulieu, E. E.,** Récentes études des protéins plasmatiques liant la testostérone, *Ann. Endocrinol.,* 29, 159, 1968.

60. **Gueriguian, J. L. and Pearlman, W.,** Some properties of a testosterone binding component of human pregnancy serum, *J. Biol. Chem.,* 243, 5226, 1968.

61. **Kato, T. and Horton, R.,** Studies of testosterone binding globulin, *J. Clin. Endocrinol.,* 28, 1160, 1968.

62. **Rosenfield, R. L.,** Relationship of androgens to female hirsutism and infertility, *J. Reprod. Med.,* 11, 87, 1973.

63. **Vermeulen, A., Stoica, T., and Verdonck, L.,** The apparent free testosterone concentration, an index of androgenicity, *J. Clin. Endocrinol.,* 33, 759, 1971.

64. **Dennis, M., Horst, H. J., Kreig, M., and Voigt, K. D.,** Plasma sex hormone-binding glubulin binding capacity in benign prostatic hypertrophy and prostatic carcinoma: comparison with an age-dependent rise in normal human males, *Acta Endocrinol., (Copenhagen),* 84, 207, 1977.

65. **Bartsch, W., Horst, H. J., Becker, H., and Nehse, G.,** Sex hormone binding globulin capacity, testosterone, 5α-dihydrotestosterone, oestradiol and prolactin in plasma of patients with prostatic carcinoma under various types of hormonal treatment, *Acta Endocrinol. (Copenhagen),* 85, 650, 1977.

66. **Baker, H. W. G., Burger, H. G., de Kretser, D. M., Hudson, B., O'Conner, S., Wang, C., Mirovics, A., Court, J., Dunlop, M., and Rennie, G. C.,** Changes in the pituitary-testicular system with age, *Clin. Endocrinol.,* 5, 349, 1976.

67. **Pirke, K. M. and Doerr, P.,** Age related changes in free plasma testosterone, dihydrotestosterone and oestradiol, *Acta Endocrinol., (Copenhagen), Suppl.,* 193, 57, 1975.

68. Farnsworth, W. E., The normal prostate and its endocrine control, in *Some Aspects of the Aetiology and Biochemistry of Prostatic Cancer,* 3rd Tenovus Workshop, Griffiths, K. and Pierrepoint, C. G., Eds., Alpha Omega Alpha, Cardiff, 1970, 3.

69. Vermeulen, A. and Verdonck, L., Some studies on the biological significance of free testosterone, *J. Steroid Biochem.,* 3, 421, 1972.

70. Lasnitzki, I. and Franklin, H. R., The influence of serum on the uptake, conversion and action of dihydrotestosterone in rat prostate glands in organ culture, *J. Endocrinol.,* 64, 289, 1975.

71. Voigt, K. D., Horst, H. J., and Kreig, M., Androgen metabolism in patients with benign prostatic hypertrophy, *Vitam. Horm. (N.Y.),* 33, 417, 1975.

72. Baird, D. T., Uno, A., and Melby, J. C., Adrenal secretion of androgens and oestrogens, *J. Endocrinol.,* 45, 135, 1969.

73. Bruchovsky, N. and Wilson, J. D., The conversion of testosterone to 5α-androstan-17β-ol-3-one by rat prostate in vivo and in vitro, *J. Biol. Chem.,* 243, 2012, 1968.

74. Bruchovsky, N. and Wilson, J. D., The intranuclear binding of testosterone and 5α androstan 17β ol-3-one by rat prostate, *J. Biol. Chem.,* 243, 5953, 1968.

75. Anderson, K. M. and Liao, S., Selective retention of dihydrotestosterone by prostatic nuclei, *Nature (London),* 219, 277, 1968.

76. Mainwaring, W. I. P., The binding of [1,2-³H]testosterone within nuclei of the rat prostate, *J. Endocrinol.,* 44, 323, 1969.

77. Farnsworth, W. E. and Brown, J. R., Metabolism of testosterone by the human prostate, *JAMA,* 183, 436, 1963.

78. Harper, M. E., Pierrepoint, C. G., Fahmy, A. R., and Griffiths, K., The metabolism of steroids in the canine prostate and testes, *J. Endocrinol.,* 49, 213, 1971.

79. Ofner, P., Effects and metabolism of hormones in normal and neoplastic prostate tissue, *Vitam. Horm. (N.Y.),* 26, 237, 1969.

80. Harper, M. E., Pike, A., Peeling, W. B., and Griffiths, K., Steroids of adrenal origin metabolised by human prostatic tissue in vivo and in vitro, *J. Endocrinol.,* 60, 117, 1974.

81. Pike, A., Peeling, W. B., Harper, M. E., Pierrepoint, C. G., and Griffiths, K., Testosterone metabolism in vivo by human prostatic tissue, *Biochem. J.,* 120, 443, 1970.

82. Becker, H., Kaufmann, J., Klosterhalfen, H., and Voigt, K. D., In vivo uptake and metabolism of [³H]testosterone and [³H]-5α-dihydrotestosterone by human benign prostatic hypertrophy, *Acta Endocrinol., (Copenhagen),* 71, 589, 1972.

83. Baulieu, E. E., Lasnitzki, I., and Robel, P., Metabolism of testosterone and action of metabolites on prostate glands grown in organ culture, *Nature (London),* 219, 1155, 1968.

84. Baulieu, E. E., Lasnitzki, I., and Robel, P., Testosterone, prostate gland and hormone action, *Biochem. Biophys. Res. Commun.,* 32, 575, 1968.

85. Farnsworth, W. E., The role of the steroid-sensitive cation-dependent ATPase in human prostatic tissue, *J. Endocrinol.,* 54, 375, 1972.

86. Harper, M. E., Pierrepoint, C. G., Fahmy, A. R., and Griffiths, K., The effect of prostatic metabolites of testosterone and other substances on the isolated deoxyribonucleic acid polymerase of the canine prostate, *Biochem. J.,* 119, 785, 1970.

87. Davies, P. and Griffiths, K., Hormonal effects in vitro on ribonucleic acid polymerase in nuclei isolated from human prostatic tissue, *J. Endocrinol.,* 59, 367, 1973.

88. Davies, P., Fahmy, A. R., Pierrepoint, C. G., and Griffiths, K., Hormone effects in vitro on prostatic ribonucleic acid polymerase, *Biochem. J.,* 129, 1167, 1972.

89. Verjans, H. L. and Eik Nes, K. B., Comparison of effects of C₁₉ (androstene or androstane) steroids on serum gonadotrophin concentrations and on accessory reproductive organ weights in gonadectomised adult male rats, *Acta Endocrinol. (Copenhagen),* 84, 829, 1977.

90. Verjans, H. L. and Eik-Nes, K. B., Gonadotrophin suppression by steroids in normal adult male rats, *Acta Endocrinol., (Copenhagen),* 84, 842, 1977.

91. Eik-Nes, K. B., Androgen metabolism by the perfused prostate, *Vitam. Horm. (N.Y.),* 33, 193, 1975.

92. Horst, H. J., Dennis, M., Kaufmann, J., and Voigt, K. D., In vivo uptake and metabolism of ³H-5α-androstane-3α,-17β-diol and of ³H-5α-androstane-3β,17β-diol by human prostatic hypertrophy, *Acta Endocrinol. (Copenhagen),* 79, 394, 1975.

93. Baulieu, E. E. and Robel, P., Testosterone metabolites: their receptors, metabolism and action in the rat ventral prostate, in *Some Aspects of the Aetiology and Biochemistry of Prostatic Cancer,* 3rd Tenovus Workshop, Griffiths, K. and Pierrepoint, C. G., Eds., Alpha Omega Alpha, Cardiff, 1970, 74.

94. Robel, P., Lasnitzki, I., and Baulieu, E. E., Hormone metabolism and action; testosterone and metabolites in prostate organ cultures, *Biochemie,* 53, 81, 1971.

95. Schmidt, H., Giba-Tziampiri, O., von Rotteck, G., and Voigt, K. D., Metabolism and mode of action of androgens in target tissues of male rats, *Acta Endocrinol. (Copenhagen),* 73, 599, 1973.

96. **Evans, C. R. and Pierrepoint, C. G.**, Demonstration of a specific cytosol receptor in the normal and hyperplastic canine prostate for 5α-androstane-3α,17α-diol, *J. Endocrinol.*, 64, 539, 1975.

97. **Chaisiri, N., Valotaire, Y., Evans, B. A. J., and Pierrepoint, C. G.**, Demonstration of a cytoplasmic receptor protein for oestrogens in the canine prostate gland, submitted for publication.

98. **Sinowatz, F. and Pierrepoint, C. G.**, Hormone effects on canine prostatic explants in organ culture, *J. Endocrinol.*, 72, 53, 1977.

99. **Rubens, R., Dhont, M., and Vermeulen, A.**, Further studies on Leydig cell function in old age, *J. Clin. Endocrinol.*, 39, 40, 1974.

100. **Mauvais-Jarvis, P.**, Etude du métabolisme 17-beta-hydroxylé de la testostérone en function de la differenciation sexuelle humaine, *C. R. Acad. Bulg. Sci.*, 262, 2753, 1966.

101. **Mauvais-Jarvis, P., Bercovici, J. P., and Flock, H. H.**, Influence des hormones sexuelles sur le metabolisme des androgens, *Rev. Fr. Etude. Clin. Biol.*, 14, 159, 1968.

102. **Mauvais-Jarvis, P., Bercovici, J. P., Crépy, O., and Gauthier, F.**, Studies on testosterone metabolism in subjects with testicular feminization, *J. Clin. Invest.*, 49, 31, 1970.

103. **Horton, R. and Tait, J. F.**, Androstenedione production and interconversion rates measured in peripheral blood and studies on the possible site of its conversion to testosterone, *J. Clin. Invest.*, 45, 351, 1966.

104. **Ito, T. and Horton, R.**, Dihydrotestosterone in human peripheral plasma, *J. Clin. Endocrinol.*, 31, 362, 1970.

105. **Saez, J. M., Forest, M. G., Morera, A. M., and Bertrand, J.**, Metabolic clearance rate and blood production rate of testosterone and dihydrotestosterone in normal subjects during pregnancy and in hyperthyroidism, *J. Clin. Invest.*, 51, 1226, 1972.

106. **Mahoudeau, J. A., Bardin, C. W., and Lipsett, M. B.**, The metabolic clearance rate and origin of plasma dihydrotestosterone and its conversion to 5α-androstanediols, *J. Clin. Invest.*, 50, 1338, 1971.

107. **Tremblay, R. R., Kowarski, A., Park, I. J., and Migeon, C. J.**, Blood production rate of dihydrotestosterone in the syndrome of male pseudohermaphroditism with testicular feminisation, *J. Clin. Endocrinol.*, 35, 101, 1972.

108. **Tremblay, R. R., Foley, T. P., Comol, P., Park, I. J., Kowarski, A., Blizzard, R. M., Jones, H. W., and Migeon, C. J.**, Plasma concentration of testosterone, dihydrotestosterone, testosterone-oestradiol binding globulin, and pituitary gonadotrophins in the syndrome of male pseudo-hermaphroditism with testicular feminisation, *Acta Endocrinol. (Copenhagen)*, 70, 331, 1972.

109. **Barberia, J., Hsieh, P., Cosgrove, M. T., and Horton, R.**, Altered blood androgens in men with prostatic hyperplasia, *Clin. Res.*, 23 (Abstr.), 233, 1975.

110. **Giorgi, E. P., Shirley, I. M., Grant, J. K., and Stewart, J. C.**, Androgen dynamics in vitro in the human prostate gland, *Biochem. J.*, 132, 465, 1973.

111. **Boyns, A. R., Griffiths, K., Pierrepoint, C. G., and Peeling, W. B.**, Prolactin and the prostate, in *Normal and Abnormal Growth of the Prostate*, Goland, M., Ed., Charles C Thomas, Springfield, Ill., 1975, 431.

112. **Farnsworth, W. E.**, Physiology and biochemistry, in *Scientific Foundations of Urology*, Vol. II, Williams, D. I. and Chisholm, G. D., Eds., Year Book Medical Publishing, Chicago, 1976, 126.

113. **King, R. J. B. and Mainwaring, W. I. P., Eds.**, *Steroid-cell Interactions*, Butterworths, London, 1974.

114. **Pirke, K. M. and Doerr, P.**, Plasma dihydrotestosterone in normal adult males and its relation to testosterone, *Acta Endocrinol., (Copenhagen)*, 79, 357, 1975.

115. **Lewis, J. G., Ghanadian, R., and Chisholm, G. D.**, Age related changes in serum 5α-dihydrotestosterone and testosterone in normal men, *J. Endocrinol.*, 67, 15P, 1975.

116. **Vermeulen, A.**, Testosterone and 5α-androstan-17β-ol-3-one (DHT) levels in man, *Acta Endocrinol. (Copenhagen)*, 83, 651, 1976.

117. **Shimazaki, J., Kato, N., Nagai, H., Yamanaka, H., and Shida, K.**, 3α-Reduction of 5α-dihydrotestosterone by rat ventral prostate, *Endocrinol., Jpn.*, 19, 97, 1972.

118. **Moore, R. J. and Wilson, J. D.**, The effect of androgenic hormones on the reduced nicotinamide adenine dinucleotide phosphate: Δ⁴-3-ketosteroid 5α-oxidoreductase of rat ventral prostate, *Endocrinology*, 93, 581, 1973.

119. **Kitay, J. I., Coyne, M. D., and Swygert, N. H.**, Influence of gonadectomy and replacement with estradiol and testosterone on formation of 5α-reduced metabolites of corticosterone by the adrenal gland of the rat, *Endocrinology*, 87, 1257, 1970.

120. **Kniewald, Z. and Milkovic, S.**, Testosterone: a regulator of 5α-reductase activity in the pituitary of male and female rats, *Endocrinology*, 92, 1772, 1973.

121. **Eik-Nes, K. B.**, An effect of isoproterenol on rates of synthesis and secretion of testosterone, *Am. J. Physiol.*, 217, 1764, 1969.

122. **Haltmeyer, G. C. and Eik-Nes, K. B.**, Production and secretion of 5α-dihydrotestosterone by the canine prostate, *Acta Endocrinol. (Copenhagen)*, 69, 394, 1972.

123. **Schlotthauer, C. F.,** Observations on the prostate gland of the dog, *J. Am. Vet. Med. Assoc.,* 81, 645, 1932.

124. **Zuckerman, S. and Groome, J. R.,** The aetiology of benign enlargement of the prostate in the dog, *J. Pathol. Bact.,* 44, 113, 1937.

125. **Smith, H. A., Jones, T. C., and Hunt, R. D., Eds.,** *Veterinary Pathology,* 4th ed., Lea & Febiger, Philadelphia, 1972.

126. **Berg, O. A.,** Parenchymatous hypertrophy of the canine prostate gland, *Acta Endocrinol. (Copenhagen),* 27, 140, 1958.

127. **Evans, C. R. and Pierrepoint, C. G.,** The effects of protein-steroid complexes on canine prostatic RNA polymerase, *Andrologia,* 8, 83, 1976.

128. **Evans, C. R. and Pierrepoint, C. G.,** Studies on the uptake and binding of 5α-androstane-3α,17α-diol by canine prostatic nuclei, *J. Endocrinol.,* 70, 31, 1976.

129. **Lacassagne, A.,** Métaplasie épidermoide de la prostate provoquée chez la souris, par des injections répétées de fortes doses de folliculine, *C. R. Seances Soc. Biol. Paris,* 113, 590, 1933.

130. **Korenchevsky, V. and Dennison, M.,** Effect of oestrone on normal and castrated male rats, *Biochem. J.,* 28, 1474, 1934.

131. **De Jongh, S. E.,** Der-einfluss von gesohlechtshormonen auf die prostate and ihre umgeburg bei der Maus, *Acta Brevia Neerl. Physiol. Pharmacol. Microbiol.,* 5, 28, 1935.

132. **Burrows, H.,** The localisation of response to oestrogenic compounds in the organs of male mice, *J. Pathol.,* 51, 423, 1935.

133. **Walsh, P. C. and Wilson, J. D.,** The induction of prostatic hypertrophy in the dog with androstanediol, *J. Clin. Invest.,* 57, 1093, 1976.

134. **Brandes, D., Kirchheim, D., and Scott, W. W.,** Ultrastructure of human prostate: normal and neoplastic, *Lab. Invest.,* 13, 1541, 1964.

135. **Kirchheim, D. and Bacon, R. L.,** Ultrastructural studies of carcinoma of the human prostate gland, *Invest. Urol.,* 6, 611, 1969.

136. **Dunning, W. F.,** Prostate cancer in the rat, *Natl. Cancer Inst. Monogr.,* 12, 351, 1963.

137. **Pollard, M.,** Spontaneous prostate adenocarcinomas in aged germfree Wistar rats, *J. Natl. Cancer Inst.,* 51, 1235, 1973.

138. **Burrows, H. and Kennaway, N. M.,** On some effects produced by applying estrin to the skin of mice, *Am. J. Cancer,* 20, 48, 1934.

139. **Fingerhut, B. and Veenema, R. J.,** Histology and radioautography of induced benign enlargement of the mouse prostate, *Invest. Urol.,* 4, 112, 1966.

140. **Walsh, P. C.,** Experimental approaches to benign prostatic hypertrophy: animal models utilizing the dog, rat and mouse, in *Benign Prostatic Hyperplasia,* Grayhack, J. T., Wilson, J. D., and Scherbenske, M. J., Eds., National Institute of Health, Bethesda, Md., 1975, 215.

141. **Harper, M. E., Peeling, W. B., Cowley, T., Brownsey, B. G., Phillips, M. E. A., Groom, G., Fahmy, D. R., and Griffiths, K.,** Plasma steroid and protein hormone concentrations in patients with prostatic carcinoma before and during oestrogen therapy, *Acta Endocrinol., (Copenhagen),* 81, 409, 1976.

142. **Asano, M.,** Studies on urinary prolactin with special reference to carcinoma of the prostate, *Jpn. J. Urol.,* 53, 901, 1962.

143. **Moon, K. H. and Flocks, R. H.,** Hormones and prostatic disease, *Urol. Dig.,* 9, 14, 1970.

144. **Isurugi, K.,** Plasma testosterone production rates in patients with prostatic cancer and benign prostatic hypertrophy, *J. Urol.,* 97, 903, 1967.

145. **Gandy, H. M. and Peterson, R. E.,** Measurement of testosterone and 17-ketosteroids in plasma by the double isotope dilution derivative technique, *J. Clin. Endocrinol.,* 28, 948, 1968.

146. **Marmorston, J., Lombardo, L. J., Myers, S. M., Gierson, M., Stern, E., and Hopkins, C. E.,** Urinary excretion of estrone and estriol by patients with prostatic cancer and benign prostatic hypertrophy, *J. Urol.,* 93, 287, 1965.

147. **Laurence, D. M. and Landau, R. L.,** Impaired ventral prostate affinity for testosterone in hypophysectomised rats, *Endocrinology,* 73, 1119, 1965.

148. **Gunn, S. A., Gould, T. C., and Anderson, W. A. D.,** The effect of growth hormone injections and prolactin preparations on the control of interstitial cell-stimulating hormone uptake, *J. Endocrinol.,* 32, 205, 1965.

149. **Asano, M.,** Basic experimental studies of the pituitary-prolactin-prostate interrelationships, *J. Urol.,* 93, 87, 1965.

150. **Huggins, C. and Russell, P. S.,** Quantitative effects of hypophysectomy on testis and prostate of dogs, *Endocrinology,* 39, 1, 1946.

151. **Lostroh, A. J. and Li, C. H.,** Stimulation of the sex accessories of hypophysectomised male rat by non-gonadotrophin hormone of the pituitary gland, *Acta Endocrinol. (Copenhagen),* 25, 1, 1957.

152. **Tullner, W. W.,** Hormonal factors in the adrenal-dependent growth of the rat ventral prostate, *Natl. Cancer Inst. Monogr.,* 12, 211, 1963.

153. **Grayhack, J. T. and Lebowitz, J. M.,** Effect of prolactin on citric acid of lateral lobe of prostate of Sprague-Dawley rat, *Invest. Urol.,* 5, 87, 1967.

154. **Chase, M. D., Geschwind, I. I., and Bern, H. A.,** Synergistic role of prolactin in response of male rat sex accessories to androgen, *Proc. Soc. Exp. Biol. Med.,* 94, 680, 1957.

155. **Wilson, D. W. and Tan, S. E.,** in *Tumour Markers: Determination and Clinical Significance,* Sixth Tenovus Workshop, Griffiths, K., Pierrepoint, C. G., and Neville, A. M., Eds., Alpha Omega Alpha, Cardiff, 1978, 341.

156. **Wilson, D. W., Griffiths, K., Nix, A. B. J., and Kemp, K. W.,** Quality control analysis in radioimmunoassays, *J. Endocrinol.,* 73, 15, 1977.

157. **Kemp, K. W., Nix, A. B. J., Wilson, D. W., and Griffiths, K.,** Internal quality control of radioimmunoassays, *J. Endocrinol.,* 76, 203, 1978.

158. **Wilson, D. W., Nix, A. B. J., Kemp, K. W., and Griffiths, K.,** Diagnostic features of internal quality control techniques in radioimmunoassay, *J. Endocrinol.,* in press.

159. **Chisholm, G. D.,** in *The Treatment of Prostatic Hypertrophy and Neoplasia,* Castro, J. E., Ed., Medical and Technical Publishing, Lancaster, 1974, 121.

160. **The British Prostate Study Group,** Multivariate analysis of plasma hormone concentrations in relation to clinical staging in patients with prostatic cancer, *Acta Endocrinol. (Copenhagen),* in press.

161. **Morfin, R. F., Leav, I., Charles, J. F., and Cavazos, L. F.,** Correlative study of morphology and C_{19}-steroid metabolism of benign and cancerous human prostatic tissue, *Cancer (Philadelphia),* 39, 1517, 1977.

162. **Griffiths, K., Maynard, P. V., Wilson, D. W., and Davies, P.,** Endocrine aspects of primary breast tumours, in *The Proceedings of the Second Symposium on Ablative Endocrine Surgery in Breast Cancer, Lyons,* Stoll, B. A. and Saez, S., Eds., Plenum Press, New York, 1978.

163. **Meites, J., Lu, K. H., Wuttke, W., Welsch, C. W., Nagasawa, H., and Quadri, S. D.,** Recent studies on functions and control of prolactin secretion in rats, *Recent Prog. Horm. Res.,* 28, 471, 1972.

164. **Boyns, A. R., Cole, E. N., Phillips, M. E. A., Hillier, S. G., Cameron, E. H. D., Griffiths, K., Shahmanesh, M., Feneley, R. C. L., and Hartog, M.,** Plasma prolactin, GH, LH, FSH, TSH and testosterone during treatment of prostatic carcinoma with oestrogens, *Eur. J. Cancer,* 10, 445, 1974.

165. **Harper, M. E., Danutra, V., Chandler, J. A., and Griffiths, K.,** The effect of 2-bromo-α-ergocryptine (CB154) administration on the hormone levels, organ weights, prostatic morphology and zinc concentration in the male rat, *Acta Endocrinol. (Copenhagen),* 83, 211, 1976.

166. **Billeter, E. and Flückiger, E.,** Evidence for a luteolytic function of prolactin in the intact cyclic rat using 2-Br-α-ergocryptine (CB154), *Experientia (Basel),* 27, 464, 1971.

167. **Siiteri, P. K. and Wilson, J. D.,** Dihydrotestosterone in prostatic hypertrophy. I. The formation and content of dihydrotestosterone in the hypertrophic prostate of man, *J. Clin. Invest.,* 49, 1737, 1970.

168. **Gloyna, R. E., Siiteri, P. K., and Wilson, D. D.,** Dihydrotestosterone in prostatic hypertrophy. II. The formation and content of dihydrotestosterone in the hyperplastic canine prostate and the effect of dihydrotestosterone on prostate growth in the dog, *J. Clin. Invest.,* 49, 1746, 1970.

169. **Millington, D. S.,** Determination of hormonal steroid concentrations in biological extracts by high resolution mass fragmentography, *J. Steroid Biochem.,* 6, 239, 1975.

170. **Millington, D. S., Buoy, M. E., Brooks, G., Harper, M. E., and Griffiths, K.,** Thin layer chromatography and high resolution selected ion monitoring for the analysis of C_{19}-steroids in human hyperplastic prostate tissue, *Biomed. Mass. Spectrom.,* 2, 219, 1975.

171. **Geller, J., Albert, J., Lopez, D., Geller, S., and Niwayama, G.,** Comparison of androgen metabolites in benign prostatic hypertrophy (BPH) and normal prostate, *J. Clin. Endocrinol.,* 43, 686, 1976.

172. **Jacobi, G. H. and Wilson, J. D.,** The formation of 5α-androstane-3α,17β-diol by dog prostate, *Endocrinology,* 99, 602, 1976.

173. **Bruchovsky, N.,** Comparison of the metabolites found in rat prostate following the in vivo administration of seven natural androgens, *Endocrinology,* 89, 1212, 1971.

174. **Lubicz-Nawrocki, C. M.,** The effect of metabolites of testosterone on the viability of hamster epididymal spermatozoa, *Endocrinology,* 58, 193, 1973.

175. **Tveter, K. J. and Aakvaag, A.,** Uptake and metabolism in vivo of testosterone-1,2-³H by accessory sex organs of male rats: influence of some hormonal compounds, *Endocrinology,* 85, 683, 1969.

176. **Giorgi, E. P., Moses, T. F., Grant, J. K., Scott, R., and Sinclair, J.,** In vitro studies of the regulation of androgen-tissue relationship in normal canine and hyperplastic human prostate, *Mol. Cell Endocrinol.,* 1, 271, 1974.

177. **Farnsworth, W. E.,** A direct effect of estrogens on prostatic metabolism of testosterone, *Invest. Urol.,* 6, 423, 1969.

178. **Groom, M., Harper, M. E., Fahmy, A. R., Pierrepoint, C. G., and Griffiths, K.,** The effect of oestrogen on the prostatic metabolism of testosterone in tissue culture, *Biochem. J.,* 122, 125, 1971.

179. Shimazaki, J., Kirihara, H., Yoshikazu, I., and Shida, K., Testosterone metabolism in the prostate; formation of androstan-17βol-3-one and androst-4-ene-3,17-dione and inhibitory effects of natural and synthetic estrogens, *Gunma J. Med. Sci.*, 14, 313, 1965.

180. Leav, I., Morfin, R. F., Ofner, P., Cavazos, L. F., and Leeds, E. B., Estrogen and castration-induced effects on canine prostate fine structure and C_{19}-steroid metabolism, *Endocrinology*, 89, 465, 1971.

181. Danutra, V., Harper, M. E., and Griffiths, K., The effect of stilboestrol analogues on the metabolism of steroids by the testes and the prostate of the rat in vitro, *J. Endocrinol.*, 59, 539, 1973.

182. Alder, A., Burger, H. G., Davis, J., Dulmanis, A., Hudson, B., Sarfaty, G., and Straffon, W. G., Carcinoma of prostate: response of plasma luteinising hormone and testosterone to oestrogen therapy, *Br. Med. J.*, 1, 28, 1968.

183. Geller, J., Baron, A., and Kleinman, S., Pituitary luteinizing hormone reserve in elderly men with prostatic disease, *J. Endocrinol.*, 48, 289, 1970.

184. Boyar, R. M., Finkelstein, J., Roffwarg, H. P., Kapen, S., Weitzman, E., and Hellman, L., Synchronisation of augmented luteinizing hormone secretion with sleep during puberty, *N. Engl. J. Med.*, 287, 582, 1973.

185. Judd, H. L., Parker, D. C., Siler, T. M., and Yen, S. S. C., The nocturnal rise of plasma testosterone in pubertal boys, *J. Clin. Endocrinol.*, 38, 710, 1974.

186. Boyar, R. M., Rosenfeld, R. S., Kapen, S., Finkelstein, J. W., Roffwarg, H. P., Weitzman, E. D., and Hellman, L., Human puberty. Simultaneous augmented secretion of luteinizing hormone and testosterone during sleep, *J. Clin. Invest.*, 54, 609, 1974.

187. Boyar, R. M., Finkelstein, J. W., David, R., and Roffwarg, H. P., Twenty-four hour patterns of plasma luteinizing hormone and follicle stimulating hormone in sexual precocity, *N. Engl. J. Med.*, 289, 282, 1973.

188. Boyar, R. M., Finkelstein, J. W., Roffwarg, H. P., Kapen, S., Weitzman, E. D., and Hellman, L., Twenty-four hour luteinizing hormone and follicle stimulating hormone secretory patterns in gonadal dysgenesis, *J. Clin. Endocrinol.*, 37, 521, 1973.

189. Rubin, R. T., Kales, A., Adler, R., Fagin, T., and Odell, W., Gonadotropin secretion during sleep in normal adult men, *Science*, 175, 196, 1972.

190. Isurugi, K., Fukutani, K., Takayasu, H., Wakabayashi, K., and Tamaoki, B. I., Age-related changes in serum luteinizing hormone (LH) and follicle stimulating hormone (FSH) levels in normal men, *J. Clin. Endocrinol.*, 399, 955, 1974.

191. Lipsett, M. B., Wilson, H., Kirschner, M. A., Korenman, S. G., Fishman, L. H., Sarfaty, G. A., and Bardin, C. W., Studies on leydig cell physiology and pathology: secretion and metabolism of testosterone, *Rec. Prog. Horm. Res.*, 22, 245, 1966.

192. Paulsen, C. A., Gordon, D. L., Carpenter, R. W., Gandy, H. M., and Drucker, W. D., Klinefelter's syndrome and its variants: a hormonal and chromosomal study, *Rec. Prog. Horm. Res.*, 24, 321, 1968.

193. Frick, J. and Kincl, F. A., The measurement of plasma testosterone by competitive protein-binding assay, *Steroids*, 13, 495, 1969.

194. Longcope, C., The effect of human chorionic gonadotrophins on plasma steroid levels in young and old men, *Steroids*, 21, 583, 1973.

195. Haug, E., Aakvaag, A., Sandt, T., and Torjesen, P. A., The gonadotrophin response to synthetic gonadotrophin releasing hormone in males in relation to age, dose and basal serum levels of testosterone, oestradiol-17β and gonadotrophins, *Acta Endocrinol. (Copenhagen)*, 77, 625, 1974.

196. Wide, L., Nillius, S. J., Gemzell, C., and Roos, P., Radioimmunosorbent assay of follicle-stimulating hormone and luteinizing hormone in serum and urine from men and women, *Acta Endocrinol. (Copenhagen) Suppl.*, 174, 1, 1973.

197. Hashimoto, T., Miyai, K., Izumi, K., and Kumahara, Y., Gonadotrophin response to synthetic LH-RH in normal subjects: correlation between LH and FSH, *J. Clin. Endocrinol.*, 37, 910, 1973.

198. Jones, G. E. and Boyns, A. R., Effect of gonadal steroids on the pituitary responsiveness to synthetic luteinizing hormone-releasing hormone in the male dog, *J. Endocrinol.*, 61, 123, 1974.

199. Jones, G. E. and Boyns, A. R., Inhibition by oestradiol of the pituitary response to luteinizing hormone releasing hormone in the dog, *J. Endocrinol.*, 68, 475, 1976.

200. Cole, E. N., Llewelyn, H., Link, J., and Boyns, A. R., Acute modulation of pituitary gonadotrophin secretion by oestradiol and testosterone in healthy men, *J. Endocrinol.*, 63, 251, 1974.

201. Samuels, L. T., Short, J. G., and Huseby, R. A., The effect of diethylstilboestrol on testicular 17α-hydroxylase and 17-desmolase activities in BALB/c mice, *Acta Endocrinol. (Copenhagen)*, 45, 487, 1964.

202. Oshima, M., Wakabayashi, K., and Tamaoki, B., The effect of synthetic oestrogen upon the biosynthesis in vitro of androgen and luteinizing hormone in the rat, *Biochim. Biophys. Acta*, 137, 356, 1967.

203. **Danutra, V., Harper, M. E., Boyns, A. R., Cole, E. N., Brownsey, B. G., and Griffiths, K.,** The effect of certain stilboestrol analogues on plasma prolactin and testosterone in the rat, *J. Endocrinol.,* 57, 207, 1973.

204. **Slaunwhite, W. R., Sandberg, A. A., Jackson, J. E., and Staubitz, W. J.,** Effects of oestrogen and HCG on androgen synthesis by human testes, *J. Clin. Endocrinol.,* 22, 992, 1962.

205. **de Jong, F. H., Hilenbroek, J. Th. J., and van der Molen, H. J.,** Oestradiol-17β, testosterone and gonadotrophins in oestradiol-17β-treated intact adult male rats, *J. Endocrinol.,* 65, 281, 1974.

206. **Harbitz, T. B.,** Morphometric studies of the Leydig cells in elderly men with spenial reference to the histology of the prostate. An analysis in an autopsy series, *Acta Pathol. Microbiol. Scand.,* 81, 301, 1973.

207. **MacLeod, R. M. and Lehmeyer, J. E.,** Studies on the mechanism of the dopamine-mediated inhibition of prolactin secretion, *Endocrinology,* 94, 1077, 1974.

208. **Jacobs, L. S., Snyder, P. J., Utiger, R. D., and Daughaday, W. H.,** Prolactin response to thyrotropin-releasing hormone in normal subjects, *J. Clin. Endocrinol.,* 36, 1069, 1973.

209. **Yamaji, T., Shimamoto, K., Ishibashi, M., Kosaka, K., and Orimo, H.,** Effect of age and sex on circulating and pituitary prolactin levels in human, *Acta Endocrinol., (Copenhagen),* 71, 83, 1976.

210. **Aragona, C. and Friesen, H.,** Specific prolactin binding sites in the prostate and testis of rats, *Endocrinology,* 97, 677, 1975.

211. **Hafiez, A. A., Lloyd, C. W., and Bartke, A.,** The role of prolactin in the regulation of testis function: the effects of prolactin and luteinising hormone on the plasma levels of testosterone and androstenedione in hypophysectomized rats, *J. Endocrinol.,* 52, 327, 1972.

212. **Hafiez, A. A., Bartke, A., and Lloyd, C. W.,** The role of prolactin in the regulation of testis function: the synergistic effects of prolactin and luteinising hormone on the incorporation of [1-¹⁴C] acetate into testosterone and cholesterol by testes from hypophysectomized rats in vitro, *J. Endocrinol.,* 53, 223, 1972.

213. **Katongole, C. B., Naftolin, F., and Short, R. V.,** Relationship between blood levels of luteinising hormone and testosterone in bulls, and the effects of sexual stimulation, *J. Endocrinol.,* 50, 457, 1971.

214. **Murray, M. A. F. and Corker, C. S.,** Levels of testosterone and luteinising hormone in plasma samples taken at 10 minute intervals in normal men, *J. Endocrinol.,* 56, 157, 1973.

215. **Rubin, R. T., Poland, R. E., and Tower, B. B.,** Prolactin-related testosterone secretion in normal adult men, *J. Clin. Endocrinol.,* 42, 112, 1976.

216. **Rubin, R. T., Gouin, P. R., Lubin, A., Poland, R. E., and Pirke, K. M.,** Nocturnal increase of plasma testosterone in men: relation to gonadotrophins and prolactin, *J. Clin. Endocrinol.,* 40, 1027, 1975.

217. **Ambrosi, B., Travaglini, P., Beck-Peccoz, P., Bara, R., Elli, R., Paracchi, A., and Faglia, G.,** Effect of sulpiride-induced hyperprolactinemia on serum testosterone response to HCG in normal men, *J. Clin. Endocrinol.,* 43, 700, 1976.

218. **Friesen, H. and Hwang, P.,** Human prolactin, *Ann. Rev. Med.,* 24, 251, 1973.

219. **Thorner, M. O., McNeilly, A. S., Hagan, C., and Besser, G. M.,** Long term treatment of galactorrhea and hypogonadism with bromocriptine, *Br. Med. J.,* 2, 419, 1974.

220. **Fang, V. S., Refetoff, S., and Rosenfield, R. L.,** Hypogonadism induced by a transplantable, prolactin-producing tumour in male rats: hormonal and morphological studies, *Endocrinology,* 95, 991, 1974.

221. **Pierrepoint, C. G., John, B. M., Groom, G. V., Wilson, D. W., and Gow, J. G.,** Prolactin and testosterone levels in plasma of fertile and infertile men, *J. Endocrinol.,* 76, 171, 1978.

222. **Kledzik, G. S., Marshall, S., Campbell, G. A., Gelato, M., and Meites, J.,** Effects of castration, testosterone, estradiol and prolactin on specific prolactin-binding activity in ventral prostate of male rats, *Endocrinology,* 98, 373, 1976.

223. **Posner, B. I., Kelly, P. A., Shiu, R. P. C., and Friesen, H. G.,** Studies of insulin, growth hormone and prolactin binding: tissue distribution, species variation and characterisation, *Endocrinology,* 95, 521, 1974.

224. **Posner, B. I., Kelly, P. A., and Friesen, H. G.,** Induction of a lactogenic receptor in rat liver: influence of estrogen and the pituitary, *Proc. Natl. Acad. Sci. U.S.A.,* 71, 2407, 1974.

225. **Posner, B. I., Kelly, P. A., and Friesen, H. G.,** Induction by a polypeptide hormone of its own receptor, *Clin. Res.,* 22, Abstr. 733, 1974.

226. **Aragona, C. and Friesen, H. G.,** Prolactin and aging, in *Benign Prostatic Hypertrophy,* Grayhack, J. T., Wilson, J. D., and Scherbenske, M. J., Eds., National Institutes of Health, Bethesda, Md., 1975, 165.

227. **Asano, M., Kanzaki, S., Sekiguchi, E., and Tasaka, T.,** Inhibition of prostatic growth in rabbits with anti-ovine prolactin serum, *J. Urol.,* 106, 248, 1971.

228. Farnsworth, W. E., Role of lactogen in prostatic physiology, *Urol. Res.*, 3, 129, 1975.

229. Lloyd, J. W., Thomas, J. A., and Mawhinney, M. G., A difference in the in vitro accumulation and metabolism of testosterone-1,2-^{3}H by the rat prostate gland following incubation with ovine or bovine prolactin, *Steroids*, 22, 473, 1973.

230. Grayhack, J. T., Bunce, P. L., Kearns, J. W., and Scott, W. W., Influence of the pituitary on prostatic response to androgen in the rat, *Bull. Johns Hopkins Hosp.*, 96, 154, 1955.

231. Skinner, J. D. and Rowson, L. E. A., Effects of unilateral cryptorchidism on sexual development in the pubescent male animal, *J. Reprod. Fert.*, 14, 349, 1967.

232. Skinner, J. D. and Rowson, L. E. A., Some effects of unilateral cryptorchidism and vasectomy on sexual development of the pubescent ram and bull, *J. Endocrinol.*, 42, 311, 1968.

233. Pierrepoint, C. G. and Davies, P., The effect of vasectomy on the activity of prostatic RNA polymerase in rats, *J. Reprod. Fert.*, 35, 149, 1973.

234. Jost, A., Recherches sur la differenciation sexuelle de l'embryon de lapin. Rôle des gonades foetales dans le differenciation sexuelle somatique, *Arch. Anat. Micros. Morphol. Exp.*, 36, 271, 1947.

235. Jost, A., Problems of foetal endocrinology. The gonadal and hypophyseal hormones, *Rec. Prog. Horm. Res.*, 8, 379, 1953.

236. Pierrepoint, C. G., Davies, P., and Wilson, D. W., The role of the epididymis and ductus deferens in the direct and unilateral control of the prostate and seminal vesicles of the rat, *J. Reprod. Fert.*, 41, 413, 1974.

237. Pierrepoint, C. G., Davies, P., Millington, D., and John, B., Evidence that the deferential vein acts as a local transport system for androgen in rat and dog, *J. Reprod. Fert.*, 43, 293, 1975.

238. Lewis, M. H. and Moffat, D. B., The venous drainage of the accessory reproductive organs of the rat with special reference to prostatic metabolism, *J. Reprod. Fert.*, 42, 497, 1975.

239. Dhabuwala, C. B., Roberts, E. E., and Pierrepoint, C. G., The radiographic demonstration of the dynamic transfer of radio-opaque material from the deferential vein to the prostate in the dog, *Invest. Urol.*, in press.

240. Dhabuwala, C. B. and Pierrepoint, C. G., Venous drainage and functional control of the canine prostate gland, *J. Endocrinol.*, 75, 105, 1972.

241. Fingerhut, B. and Veenema, R. J., The effect of bilateral adrenalectomy on induced benign prostatic hyperplasia in mice, *J. Urol.*, 97, 508, 1967.

242. Tisell, L. E., Effect of cortisone on the growth of the ventral prostate, the dorsolateral prostate, the coagulating glands and the seminal vesicles in castrated, adrenalectomised and castrated non-adrenalectomised rats, *Acta Endocrinol. (Copenhagen)*, 64, 637, 1970.

243. Tisell, L. E., Adrenal effect on the growth of the ventral and dorso-lateral prostate in castrated rats injected with oestradiol, *Acta Endocrinol. (Copenhagen)*, 71, 191, 1972.

244. Muntzing, J., The androgenic action of adrenal implants in the ventral prostate of adult, castrated and oestrogen treated rats, *Acta Pharmacol. Toxicol.*, 30, 203, 1971.

245. Coyne, M. D. and Kitay, J. I., Effect of ovariectomy on pituitary secretion of ACTH, *Endocrinology*, 85, 1097, 1969.

246. Nalbanov, A. V., Ed., *Advances in Neuroendocrinology*, University of Illinois Press, Urbana, 1963.

247. von Berswordt-Wallrabe, R., Bielitz, U., Elger, W., and Steinbeck, H., Progesterone and the ventral prostate gland in juvenile rats, *J. Urol.*, 103, 180, 1970.

248. Farnsworth, W. E., Human prostatic dehydroepiandrosterone sulfate sulfatase, in *Normal and Abnormal Growth of the Prostate*, Goland, M., Ed., Charles C Thomas, Springfield, Ill., 1975, 160.

249. Rivarola, M. A., Saez, J. M., Meyer, W. J., Jenkins, M. E., and Migeon, C. J., Metabolic clearance rate and blood production rate of testosterone and androst-4-ene-3,17-dione under basal conditions, ACTH and HCG stimulation. Comparison with urinary production rate of testosterone, *J. Clin. Endocrinol.*, 26, 1208, 1966.

250. Beitens, I. Z., Bayard, F., Kowarski, A., and Migeon, C. J., The effect of ACTH administration on plasma testosterone, dihydrotestosterone and serum LH concentrations in normal men, *Steroids*, 21, 553, 1973.

251. Cowley, T. H., Brownsey, B. G., Harper, M. E., Peeling, W. B., and Griffiths, K., The effect of ACTH on plasma testosterone and androstenedione concentrations in patients with prostatic carcinoma, *Acta Endocrinol. (Copenhagen)*, 81, 310, 1976.

252. Boyns, A. R., Cole, E. N., Golder, M. P., Danutra, V., Harper, M. E., Brownsey, B. G., Cowley, T. H., Jones, G. E., and Griffiths, K., Prolactin studies with the prostate, in *Prolactin and Carcinogenesis*, Boyns, A. R. and Griffiths, K., Eds., Alpha Omega Alpha, Cardiff, 1972, 207.

253. Millington, D. S., Golder, M. P., Cowley, T. H., London, D., Roberts, H., Butt, W. R., and Griffiths, K., In vitro synthesis of steroids by a feminising adrenocortical carcinoma: effect of prolactin and other protein hormones, *Acta Endocrinol. (Copenhagen)*, 82, 561, 1976.

254. Vermeulen, A., Suy, E., and Rubens, R., Effect of prolactin on plasma DHEA (S) levels, *J. Clin. Endocrinol.*, 44, 1222, 1977.

255. Bassi, F., Giusti, G., Bansi, L., Cattaneo, S., Giannotti, P., Forti, G., Parznzagli, M., Vigiani, C., and Serio, M., Plasma androgens in women with hyperprolactinaemic amenorrhoea, *Clin. Endocrinol. (Copenhagen)*, 6, 5, 1977.

256. Boyar, R. M. and Hellman, L., Syndrome of benign nodular hyperplasia associated with feminization and hyperprolactinemia, *Ann. Int. Med.*, 80, 389, 1974.

257. Marshall, S., Kledzik, G. S., Gelato, M., Campbell, G. A., and Meites, J., Effects of estrogen and testosterone on specific prolactin binding in the kidneys and adrenals of rats, *Steroids*, 27, 187, 1976.

258. Bartke, A., Smith, M. S., Michael, S. D., Peron, F. G., and Dalterio, S., Effects of experimentally-induced chronic hyperprolactinemia on testosterone and gonadotrophin levels in male rats and mice, *Endocrinology*, 100, 182, 1977.

259. de Peretti, E. and Forest, M. G., Unconjugated dehydroepiandrosterone plasma levels in normal subjects from birth to adolescence in human: the use of sensitive ratioimmunoassays, *J. Clin. Endocrinol.*, 43, 982, 1976.

260. Bulbrook, R. D., Franks, L. M., and Greenwood, F. C., Hormone excretion in prostatic cancer: the early and late effects of endocrine treatment on urinary oestrogens, 17-ketosteroids and 17-ketogenic steroids, *Acta Endocrinol. (Copenhagen)*, 31, 481, 1959.

261. Birke, G., Franksson, C., and Plantin, L. O., On excretion of androgens in carcinoma of prostate, *Acta Endocrinol. (Copenhagen)*, 17, 17, 1954.

262. Robinson, M. R. G. and Thomas, B. S., Effect of hormonal therapy on plasma testosterone levels in prostatic carcinoma, *Br. Med. J.*, 4, 391, 1971.

263. Sciarra, F., Sorcini, D., di Silverio, F., and Gagliardi, V., Plasma testosterone and androstenedione after orchiectomy in prostatic adenocarcinoma, *Clin. Endocrinol.*, 2, 101, 1973.

264. Mainwaring, W. I. P., The mechanism of action of androgens, in *Monographs on Endocrinology*, Vol. 10, Springer-Verlag, Berlin, 1977.

265. Giorgi, E. P., Studies on androgen transport into canine prostate in vitro, *J. Endocrinol.*, 68, 109, 1976.

266. Cowan, R. A., Cowan, S. K., Giles, C. A., and Grant, J. K., Prostatic distribution of sex hormone-binding globulin and cortisol-binding globulin in benign hyperplasia, *J. Endocrinol.*, 71, 121, 1976.

267. Tveter, K. J., Some aspects of the pathogenesis of prostatic hyperplasia, *Acta Pathol. Microbiol. Scand., Sect. A., Suppl.*, 248, 167, 1974.

268. Prout, G. R., Kliman, B., Daly, J. J., McLaughlin, R. A., and Griffin, P. P., In vitro uptake of [³H]testosterone, and its conversion to dihydrotestosterone by prostatic carcinoma and other tissues, *J. Urol.*, 116, 603, 1976.

269. Habib, F. K., Lee, I. R., Stitch, S. R., and Smith, P. H., Androgen levels in the plasma and prostatic tissues of patients with benign hypertrophy and carcinoma of the prostate, *J. Endocrinol.*, 71, 99, 1976.

270. Verhoeven, G., Heyns, W., and De Moor, P., Testosterone receptors in the prostate and other tissues, *Vitam. Horm. (N. Y.)*, 33, 265, 1975.

271. Jacobi, G. H. and Wilson, J. D., Formation of 5α-androstane-3α,17β-diol by normal and hypertrophic human prostate, *J. Clin. Endocrinol.*, 44, 107, 1977.

272. Krieg, M., Bartsch, W., Herzer, S., Becker, H., and Voigt, K. D., Quantification of androgen binding, androgen tissue levels, and sex hormone binding globulin in prostate, muscle and plasma of patients with benign prostatic hypertrophy, *Acta Endocrinol., (Copenhagen)*, 86, 200, 1977.

273. Krieg, M., Dennis, M., and Voigt, K. D., Comparison between the binding of 19-nortestosterone, 5α-dihydrotestosterone and testosterone in rat prostate and bulbocavernosus/levator ani muscle, *J. Endocrinol.*, 70, 379, 1976.

274. Krieg, M., Horst, H. J., and Sterba, M. L., Binding and metabolism of 5α-androstane-3α,-17β-diol and 5α-androstane-3β,17β-diol in the prostate, seminal vesicles and plasma of male rats: studies in vivo and in vitro, *J. Endocrinol.*, 64, 529, 1975.

275. Boesel, R. W., Klipper, R. W., and Shain, S. A., Identification of limited capacity androgen binding components in nuclear and cytoplasmic fractions of canine prostate, *Endocr. Res. Commun.*, 4, 71, 1977.

276. Davies, P., Receptors in the human prostate, in *Tumour markers, Determination and Clinical Significance*, Sixth Tenovus Workshop, Griffiths, K., Pierrepoint, C. G., and Neville, A. M., Eds., Alpha Omega Alpha, Cardiff, 1978, 175.

277. Davies, P., Thomas, P., and Griffiths, K., The influence of steroid-receptor complexes on the stages of transcription of target-tissue chromatin, *J. Steroid Biochem.*, 7, 993, 1976.

278. Davies, P., Thomas, P., and Griffiths, K., Measurement of free and occupied cytoplasmic and nuclear androgen receptor sites in rat ventral prostate gland, *J. Endocrinol.*, 74, 393, 1977.

279. Davies, P. and Griffiths, K., Similarities between 5α-dihydrotestosterone-receptor complexes from human and rat prostatic tissue: effects on RNA polymerase activity, *Mol. Cell. Endocrinol.*, 3, 143, 1975.

280. **Mainwaring, W. I. P. and Milroy, E. J. G.,** Characterisation of the specific androgen receptors in the human prostate gland, *J. Endocrinol.,* 57, 371, 1973.
281. **Ghanadian, R., Chisholm, G. D., and Fotherby, K.,** Intracellular localisation of 5α-dihydrotestosterone in human benign prostatic hypertrophy, *Clin. Chim. Acta,* 73, 521, 1976.
282. **Davies, P.,** The influence of androgen-receptor complexes on transcription by rat and human prostatic ribonnucleic acid polymerases, *Biochem. Soc. Trans.,* 3, 1133, 1975.
283. **Davies, P. and Griffiths, K.,** Influence of steroid-receptor complexes on transcription by human hypertrophied prostatic RNA polymerases, *Mol. Cell. Endocrinol.,* 5, 269, 1976.
284. **Rosen, V., Jung, I., Baulieu, E. E., and Robel, P.,** Androgen-binding proteins in human benign prostatic hypertrophy, *J. Clin. Endocrinol.,* 41, 761, 1975.
285. *Estrogen Receptors in Human Breast Cancer,* McGuire, W. L., Carbone, P. P., and Vollmer, E. P., Eds., Raven Press, New York, 1975.
286. **Martini, L. and Motta, M., Eds.,** *Androgens and Antiandrogens,* Raven Press, New York, 1977.
287. **Mainwaring, W. I. P.,** in *Steroid Hormones and Cancer,* Menon, K. M. J. and Reel, J. R., Eds., Plenum Press, New York, 1976, 152.
288. **Neri, R. and Monahan, M.,** Effects of a novel nonsteroidal antiandrogen on canine prostatic hyperplasia, *Invest. Urol.,* 10, 123, 1972.
289. **Neri, R., Florance, K., Koziol., P., and Van Cleave, S.,** A biological profile of a non-steroidal antiandrogen, SCH 13521, (4′-nitro-3′-trifluoromethylisobutyrylanilide), *Endocrinology,* 91, 427, 1972.
290. **Mainwaring, W. I. P., Mangan, F. R., Feherty, P. A., and Friefeld, M.,** An investigation into the anti-androgenic properties of the non-steroidal compound, SCH 13521 (4′nitro-3′-trifluoromethylisobutyrylanilide), *Mol. Cell. Endocrinol.,* 1, 113, 1974.
291. **Wagner, R. K., Schulze, K. H., and Jungblut, P. W.,** Estrogen and androgen receptor in human prostate and prostatic tumour tissue, *Acta Endocrinol. (Copenhagen), Suppl.,* 193, (Abstr.), 52, 1975.
292. **Hawkins, E. F., Nijs, M., Brassinne, C., and Tagnon, H. J.,** Steroid receptors in the human prostate. I. Estradiol-17β binding in benign prostatic hypertrophy, *Steroids,* 26, 458, 1975.
293. **Bashirelahi, N. and Armstrong, E. G.,** 17β-Estradiol binding by human prostate, in *Normal and Abnormal Growth of the Prostate,* Goland, M., Ed., Charles C Thomas, Springfield, Ill., 1975, 632.
294. **De Klerk, D. P., Heston, W. D. W., and Coffey, D. L.,** Studies on the role of macromolecular synthesis in the growth of the prostate, in *Benign Prostatic Hyperplasia,* Grayhack, J. T., Wilson, J. D., and Scherbenske, M. J., Eds., National Institutes of Health, Bethesda, Md., 1975, 43.
295. **Cowan, R. A., Cowan, S. K., and Grant, J. K.,** Binding of methyltrienolone (R1881) to a progesterone receptor-like component of human prostate cytosol, *J. Endocrinol.,* 74, 281, 1977.
296. **Lasnitzki, I., Whitaker, R. H., and Withycombe, J. F. R.,** The effect of steroid hormones in the growth pattern and RNA synthesis in human benign prostatic hyperplasia in organ culture, *Br. J. Cancer,* 32, 168, 1975.
297. **Lasnitzki, I.,** The rat prostate in organ culture, in *Some Aspects of the Aetiology and Biochemistry of Prostatic Cancer,* Griffiths, K. and Pierrepoint, C. G., Eds., Alpha Omega Alpha, Cardiff, 1970, 68.
298. **Centifanto, Y. M., Kaufman, H. E., Zam, Z. S., Drylis, D. M., and Deardourff, S. L.,** Herpesvirus particles in prostatic carcinoma cells, *J. Virol.,* 12, 1608, 1973.
299. **Dmochowski, L., Maruyama, K., Ohtsuki, Y., Seman, G., Bowen, J. M., Newton, W. A., and Johnson, D. E.,** Virologic and immunologic studies of human prostatic carcinoma, *Cancer Chemother. Rep.,* 59, 17, 1975.
300. **Ohtsuki, Y., Seman, G., and Maruyama, K.,** Ultrastructural studies of human prostatic neoplasia, *Cancer (Philadelphia),* 37, 2295, 1976.
301. **Todaro, G. J. and Huebner, R. J.,** The viral oncogene hypothesis: new evidence, *Proc. Natl. Acad. Sci.,* 69, 1009, 1972.
302. **Rotkin, I. D.,** Studies in the epidemiology of prostatic cancer: expanded sampling, *Cancer Treat. Rep.,* 61, 173, 1977.
303. **Potts, C. L.,** Cadmium proteinuria — the health of battery workers exposed to cadmium oxide dust, *Ann. Occup. Hyg.,* 8, 55, 1965.
304. **Adams, R. G., Harrison, J. F., and Scott, P.,** The development of cadmium-induced proteinuria, impaired renal function and oesteomalacia in alkaline battery workers, *Q. J. Med.,* 38, 425, 1969.
305. **Kipling, M. D. and Waterhouse, J. A. H.,** Cadmium and prostatic carcinoma, *Lancet,* i, 730, 1962.
306. **Lemon, R. A., Lee, J. S., Wagoner, J. K., and Blejer, H. P.,** Cancer mortality among cadmium production workers, *Ann. N.Y. Acad. Sci.,* 271, 273, 1976.
307. **Aughey, E. and Scott, R.,** in discussions *Some Aspects of the Aetiology and Biochemistry of Prostatic Cancer,* Griffiths, K. and Pierrepoint, C. G., Eds., Alpha Omega Alpha, Cardiff, 1970, 145.

308. **Parizek, J. and Zahor, Z.,** Effect of cadmium salts on testicular tissue, *Nature (London)*, 177, 1036, 1956.

309. **Parizek, J.,** Sterilization of the male by cadmium salts, *J. Reprod. Fertil.*, 1, 294, 1960.

310. **Gunn, S. A., Gould, T. C., and Anderson, W. A. D.,** The selective injurious response of testicular and epididymal blood vessels to cadmium and its prevention by zinc, *Am. J. Pathol.*, 42, 685, 1963.

311. **Chiquone, A. D.,** Observations on the early events of cadmium necrosis of the testis, *Anat. Rec.*, 149, 23, 1964.

312. **Chen, R. W., Wagner, P. A., Hoekstra, W. G., and Ganther, H. E.,** Affinity labelling studies with [109]Cadmium in cadmium-induced testicular injury in rats, *J. Reprod. Fertil.*, 38, 293, 1974.

313. **Berliner, A. R. and Jones-Witters, P.,** Early effects of a lethal cadmium dose on gerbil testis, *Biol. Reprod.*, 13, 240, 1975.

314. **Gunn, S. A., Gould, T. C., and Anderson, W. A. D.,** Competition of cadmium for zinc in rat testis and dorso-lateral prostate, *Acta Endocrinol. (Copenhagen)*, 37, 24, 1961.

315. **Favino, A., Baillie, A. H., and Griffiths, K.,** Androgen synthesis by the testes and adrenal glands of rats poisoned with cadmium chloride, *J. Endocrinol.*, 35, 185, 1966.

316. **Levy, L. S., Roe, F. J. C., Malcolm, D., Kazantizis, G., Clack, J., and Platt, H. S.,** Absence of prostatic changes in rats exposed to cadmium, *Ann. Occup. Hyg.*, 16, 111, 1973.

317. **Malcolm, D.,** Potential carcinogenic effect of cadmium in animals and man, *Ann. Occup. Hyg.*, 15, 33, 1972.

318. **Chandler, J. A. and Timms, B. G.,** The effect of testosterone and cadmium on the rat lateral prostate in organ culture, *Virchows Arch. B.*, 25, 17, 1977.

319. **Timms, B. G., Chandler, J. A., Morton, M. S., and Groom, G. V.,** The effect of cadmium administration in vivo on plasma testosterone and the ultrastructure of rat lateral prostate, *Virchows Arch. B.*, 25, 33, 1977.

320. **Mawson, C. A. and Fischer, M. I.,** Zinc content of the genital organs of the rat, *Nature (London)*, 167, 859, 1951.

321. **Gunn, S. A. and Gould, T. C.,** The relative importance of androgen and oestrogen in the selective uptake of Zn^{65} by the dorso-lateral prostate of the rat, *Endocrinology*, 58, 443, 1956.

322. **Gunn, S. A. and Gould, T. C.,** Hormone inter-relationships affecting the selective uptake of ^{65}Zn by the dorso-lateral prostate of the hypophysectomized rat, *J. Endocrinol.*, 16, 18, 1957.

323. **Timms, B. G., Chandler, J. A., and Sinowatz, F.,** The ultrastructure of basal cells of rat and dog prostate, *Cell. Tissue Res.*, 173, 543, 1976.

324. **Aughey, E., Scott, R., and McLaughlin, I.,** Fine structural changes in rat prostate 5 months after the experimental introduction of 20-methylcholanthrene, *Br. J. Urol.*, 46, 561, 1974.

325. **Franks, L. M.,** Benign prostatic hyperplasia: gross and microscopic anatomy, in *Benign Prostatic Hyperplasia*, Grayhack, J. T., Wilson, J. D., and Scherbenske, M. J., Eds., National Institutes of Health, Bethesda, Md., 1975, 63.

326. **Sheppard, J. R. and Bannai, J. R.,** Cyclic AMP and cell proliferation, in *Control of Proliferation in Animal Cells*, Vol. 1, Clarkson, B. and Baserga, R., Eds., Cold Spring Harbor Laboratory, Cold Spring Harbor, N.Y., 1974, 571.

327. **Goldberg, N. D., Haddox, M. K., Dunham, E., Lopez, C., and Hadden, J. W.,** The Yin-Yang hypothesis of biological control: opposing influences of cyclic GMP and cyclic AMP in the regulation of cell proliferation and other biological processes, in *Control of Proliferation in Animal Cells*, Vol. 1, Clarkson, B. and Baserga, R., Eds., Cold Spring Harbor Laboratory, New York, 1974, 609.

328. **Williams-Ashman, H. G., Jänne, J., Coppoc, G. L., Geroch, M. E., and Schenone, A.,** New aspects of polyamine biosynthesis in eukaryotic organisms, in *Advances in Enzyme Regulation*, Vol. 10, G. Weber, G., Ed., Pergamon Press, Oxford, 1972, 225.

329. **Williams-Ashman, H. G., Corti, A., and Sheth, A. R.,** Formation and functions of aliphatic polyamines in the prostate gland and its secretions, in *Normal and Abnormal Growth of the Prostate*, Goland, M., Ed., Charles C Thomas, Springfield, 1975, 222.

330. **Fair, W. R., Clark, R. B., and Wehner, N.,** A correlation of seminal polyamine levels and semen analysis in the human, *Fertil. Steril.*, 23, 38, 1972.

331. **Bachrach, V.,** *Functions of Naturally Occurring Polyamines*, Academic Press, New York, 1973.

332. **Stevens, L.,** The biochemical role of naturally occurring polyamines in nucleic acid synthesis, *Biol. Rev.*, 45, 1, 1970.

333. **Tabor, H. and Tabor, C. W.,** Biosynthesis and metabolism of 1,4-diaminobutane, spermine, spermidine and related amines, *Adv. Enzymol.*, 36, 203, 1972.

334. **Williams-Ashman, W. G., Coppoc, G. L., and Weber, G.,** Imbalance in ornithine metabolism in hepatomas of different growth rates as expressed in formation of putrescine, spermidine and spermine, *Cancer Res.*, 32, 1924, 1972.

335. **Russell, D. H.,** The roles of the polyamines, putrescine, spermidine and spermine in normal and malignant tissues, *Life Sci.*, 13, 1635, 1973.

336. **Russell, D. H.,** Polyamines as markers of tumour kinetics, in *Tumour Markers: Determination and Clinical Role,* Griffiths, K., Pierrepoint, C. G., and Neville, A. M., Eds., Alpha Omega Alpha, Cardiff, 1978.

337. **MacMahon, B., Cole, P., Lin, T. M., Lowe, C. R., Mirra, A. P., Ravnihar, B., Salber, E. J., Valaoras, V. G., and Yuasa, S.,** Age at first birth and breast cancer risk, *Bull. W.H.O.,* 43, 209, 1970.

338. **Chaisiri, N. and Pierrepoint, C. G.,** Demonstration of differences in receptor site concentration for oestrogens in separated epithelial and stromal fractions of the canine prostate, *J. Endocrinol.* in press.

339. **Harper, M. E.,** unpublished data.

Chapter 2

HORMONAL THERAPY OF PROSTATIC CANCER

Clarence V. Hodges

TABLE OF CONTENTS

I. INTRODUCTION

Carcinoma of the prostate gland is one of the most common tumors of the adult male, ranking behind lung and colorectal cancer. Over 19,000 died of this affliction and there were 57,000 new cases diagnosed in 1977 in the U.S.[1]

In patients with prostatic cancer, staged according to Whitmore's[2] classification, less than 10% will be Stage A, confined to the prostate gland and detectible only on histo-pathologic study, or stage B, a palpable nodule occupying some or most of the prostate gland, but still confined to it. Stages A and B make up about 20 to 25% of prostatic cancers at the time of presentation and are the only stages in which there is reasonable hope of cure by surgical extirpation. Stage C, in which there is spread outside the prostate gland, but confined within the pelvis, makes up about 40% of prostatic cancers at the time of clinical diagnosis. These may be treated by radiation, although if there is spread to pelvic lymph nodes as occurs in 40 to 50%,[3] the prognosis is poor.

Stage D tumors are those which have spread to lymph nodes, to bones, or to other parts of the body. These are the tumors with which we shall be concerned in this chapter; they make up 35 to 40% of the total group.

II. HISTORICAL

Langstaff[4] in 1817 identified and reported an authentic case of prostatic cancer. Thompson[5] reported the first large series of prostatic cancers, 23 cases, in 1858. White[6] in 1895 reported a series of 111 patients who underwent orchiectomy for symptoms of marked prostatic obstruction with large amounts of residual urine. His thesis was that enlargement of the prostate bears the same relationship to the testes as fibroid disease in the uterus does to the ovaries. Bilateral orchiectomy was carried out on all patients with overall improvement of 75%. Many of these patients were in desperate straits; the operative mortality was 18%. No distinction was made between benign and malignant enlargement; however, 4 of 111 patients were described as having an extremely hard prostate gland and these patients all improved dramatically. Cabot[7] in 1896 reviewed the evidence in White's series for the effect of castration on a large prostate, as follows: "castration would seem to be especially efficacious in cases of large tense prostates when the obstruction is due to pressure on the lateral lobes upon the urethra. Castration is of but little use in myomatous and fibrous prostates." In 1939 and 1940, Huggins and his co-workers[8,9] described the classic experiments in dogs, in which it was shown that:

- Morphologic and functional prostatic atrophy followed castration.
- Daily injections of testosterone propionate reversed the postcastrational change and reconstructed the prostate.
- In a castrate dog, whose prostatic secretion had been steadily increasing due to daily injections of testosterone propionate, and who then received increasing daily doses of stilbesterol, the characteristic rising curve of prostatic secretion became a plateau and an increased dosage of estrogen caused decrease in the amount of secretion.

Kutscher and Wolberg[10] discovered that acid phosphatase is found in the prostate of adult human males in amounts greatly in excess of those in other organs. An objective method of determining the activity of prostatic cancer was suggested when Gutman and Gutman[11] described elevation of serum acid phosphatase levels in patients with metastatic prostatic cancer. Huggins and Hodges[12] found that acid and alkaline serum phosphatase could be used to follow the course of patients who underwent castration and estrogen and androgen administration after the diagnosis of metastatic prostatic cancer had been made. They concluded that "prostatic cancer is influenced by androgenic activity in the body. At least with respect to serum phosphatases, disseminated carcinoma of the prostate is activated by androgen injections." In a subsequent paper,

Huggins, Stevens, and Hodges[13] reported that 21 consecutive patients had been treated by castration for far-advanced or metastatic carcinoma of the prostate. "Four patients died at eight months after the operation; in two cases, the operation was done too recently to allow deductions as to its efficacy and in 15 cases appreciable clinical improvement occurred. The objective evidence of benefit after orchiectomy consisted of a great decrease in the levels of serum phosphatase in all but two cases, an increase in weight (and appetite), an increase in the red cells of the peripheral blood, and decrease in the amount of pain, shrinkage of the primary lesion, increased density of the metastatic lesion, in the roentgenograms; and in one case, improvement in neurologic signs of compression of the cauda equina by metastases. Improvement was greater than we have observed in any case in which far-advanced or metastatic cancer was treated any other way. It is certain that in many cases, regression of the neoplasm is not complete."

III. DIAGNOSIS

Unfortunately, most prostatic cancers in Stages A and early B are asymptomatic and are detected only by the routine physical examination. Local symptoms are usually due to compression of the prostatic urethra by the tumor as it grows and consist of lessening of the urinary stream and frequency of and incomplete bladder emptying. Rectal prostatic palpation to the trained clinician will show an area of increased consistency, usually nontender, which must be differentiated from calculi, granulomatoses, postsurgical scarring, and adenomata. Clinical experience will refine the tactus eruditas, but only to about 50% accuracy in the smallest nodules. Histopathologic diagnosis is crucial and is obtained in most cases by transrectal or transperineal needle biopsy.

A. Staging

Accurate staging of prostatic cancer is necessary for a rational approach to therapy. In a study done at this institution,[14] of 252 Stage B patients who were selected for radical prostatectomy on the basis of rectal examination, 16% were subsequently reported by the pathologist as showing invasion of the seminal vesicle area and therefore Stage C. On skeletal bone survey, one looks for the characteristic blotchy increases in density, indicating the mixed osteoblastic (predominantly) and osteolytic activity, particularly in the pelvis, lower lumbar spine, and upper femora. The bone survey will also help to rule out arthritis and other conditions which cause uptake of technetium 99m polyphosphate when this material is used for a subsequent skeletal radionuclide scan to determine areas of increased uptake of the material. Excretory urography will indicate the possibility of obstruction of the lower ends of the ureters by prostatic cancer encroachment into the bladder floor and cystoscopy, particularly in patients with obstructive symptoms will help to define the extent of such involvement.

B. Phosphatase Serum Determinations

Enzymatic methods of determining acid and alkaline phosphatase in serum have improved over the years since 1941, but are now being replaced by more sensitive and sophisticated methods. These include the radioimmunoassay test of Cooper and Foti,[15] which appears to be accurate (but expensive) and the counterimmune electrophoresis method,[16] which appears to be cheaper, but not as sensitive. Bone marrow acid phosphatase determinations have been recommended[17] as being more sensitive than determinations made on peripheral serum, but this belief has recently been subject to serious challenge.[18]

C. Lymphangiography

Lymphangiograms by bipedal route have been used to determine whether prostatic cancer has spread to pelvic lymph nodes. In our experience it has been difficult to visualize the pelvic lymph nodes and to weed out false readings. There is a real need for new techniques that would accurately delineate the pelvic lymph nodes, particularly the obturator and hypogastric groups, since this would obviate the need for surgical staging.

D. Surgical Staging

Radical surgery is contraindicated in patients with pelvic lymph node involvement. The efficacy of radiation therapy when pelvic lymph nodes are involved is still a matter of conjecture. The need to determine the degree of involvement of pelvic lymph nodes has led to retropubic surgical staging by means of lymphadenectomy. This needs to be a thorough bilateral pelvic lymphadenectomy rather than a node palpation and plucking excursion. The morbidity of this procedure alone is not inconsiderable, consisting of lymphocele formation (10%),[19] wound infections, and leg edema.

E. Endocrine Treatment

Central issues revolve around the best time to begin endocrine treatment, the best initial endocrine therapy, i.e., the proper sequence of estrogens and orchiectomy, and considerations of the proper dosage, side effects, combinations of various agents, and the overall maintenance of comfort and life quality in an essentially incurable disease.

One of the frequently encountered problems is the elderly male in whom stage D disease is evident, but in whom no symptoms are found. Two definite schools of thought exist. Studies of the Veterans Administration Co-Operative Urologic Research Group (VACURG)[20] suggest that endocrine therapy benefits in a given patient last for a fixed period of time, after which he tends to escape from control. This has led to opinions that such patients should have no treatment until such time as symptoms become manifest, thus prolonging their enjoyable life. On the other hand, experts such as Resnick and Grayhack[21] feel that prostatic cancer should be treated as soon as it is diagnosed, but admit that their opinion may be emotional rather than rational. At our institution, we have concurred with the former group and withheld therapy until symptoms, particularly bone pain, pathologic fractures, epidural spinal cord compression, or aplastic anemia from bone marrow involvement have indicated that the disease is pursuing an active clinical course. Elevation of the serum acid phosphatase has been suggested as a reason for instituting hormonal therapy, but unless it is accompanied by one of the above symptoms, this in itself does not constitute indication for therapy.

The next controversy surrounds which agent shall be first employed, estrogens or orchiectomy. Estrogens are cheap, noninvasive, and nonmutilating. In a susceptible patient, they are rapidly effective, ameliorating pain and other symptoms within as little as 72 hr. However, they cause painful breast enlargement unless this is anticipated by radiotherapy to the breast or bilateral simple mastectomy. In the case of stilbesterol, which is the commonly used estrogen, doses of 5 mg/day were associated in the first VACURG study,[20] with increased incidence of heart disease and cerebro-vascular accidents. This caused the stilbesterol series and the stilbesterol-orchiectomy combination to be associated with poorer survival than either the orchiectomy or the placebo groups. In addition to these problems, estrogen administration in some males results in marked depression and loss of well being, which is quite dramatic and may be associated with only one type of all types of estrogens. Estrogens also depend on patient compliance, a trust that is often misplaced.

Orchiectomy is a simple procedure of no mortality and very little morbidity. It is permanent and does not depend on patient compliance for effect. It is, however, mutilating, invasive, and harmful to the patient's self image.

IV. MECHANISMS OF HORMONAL ACTION

A. Bilateral Orchiectomy

Bilateral orchiectomy in the adult male removes the source of over 90% of his testosterone, the total of which is approximately 5 to 10 mg/day.[22] The evidence for the conversion of other steroid hormones to testosterone and the formation of 5-alpha-dihydrotestosterone from testosterone in target tissues is discussed in Volume II, Chapter 1. The conclusion that "testosterone and certain of its metabolites are concerned in the control of prostatic growth and function and inner conversion of these steroids within the gland may provide a delicate regulatory mechanism for the various glandular processes" seems to be justified. The amount and functional quality of conversion of adrenal steroids into active androgens demands further study.

B. Estrogens

Estrogens are believed to play their major role by influencing the pituitary, causing it to reduce the release of luteinizing hormone. With the resulting decrease in stimulation of interstitial cells to produce testosterone, there is an ultimate loss of prostate growth and metabolism. In Volume II, Chapter 6, the possibility of a direct inhibitory action of estrogen on the testis is considered. It has also been shown by Flocks and Marberger[23] that estrogens may be deposited directly in prostatic cells and may have a local brief direct action. In the castrate dog, it has been demonstrated that stilbesterol will decrease the output of prostatic fluid that has been restored by exogenous testosterone;[9] this has also been demonstrated to be true in the castrate hypophysectomized dog.[24]

C. Stilbesterol

Stilbesterol, a synthetic, nonsteroidal hormone, is the one most commonly employed to inhibit prostatic cancer metastases. It is cheap, relatively nontoxic, and well tolerated except for gynecomastia. Most patients receiving stilbesterol are impotent, but this effect varies widely and is somewhat dose-related. Several groups[26-30] have shown that it requires stilbesterol of 3.0 mg/day or more to reduce the serum testosterone to castrate levels (below 50 ng/100 mℓ). Doses below 1.0 mg/day of stilbesterol are not effective in lowering plasma testosterone, but 1.0 mg/day has a definite effect, although not lowering this value to castrate levels. Since it is common clinical knowledge that most patients with prostatic cancer sensitive to estrogens will exhibit pronounced relief at 1.0 mg/day, considerable question is raised as to whether lowering of plasma testosterone to castrate levels is the objective of estrogen therapy or merely a concomitant. Conjugated estrogens (Premarin®) 2.5 mg three times a day and ethinyl estradiol (Estinyl®) 0.05 mg twice daily are as effective in lowering plasma testosterone as stilbesterol 3 mg/day.[30] With regard to another estrogen, chlorotrianisene (TACE®), Baker[31] has demonstrated moderate suppression of plasma testosterone levels (40 to 60%) while Schearer et al.[30] found that when chlorotrianisene was given to their group of patients, there was no significant suppression of plasma testosterone levels.

The initial studies of the Veterans Administration Co-Operative Urologic Research Group[20] showed that in each series of patients in which stilbesterol, 5 mg daily, was employed, the death rate from heart disease and cerebro-vascular accidents was higher. It is believed that this is due to suppression by estrogen of the naturally occurring fibrinolysins, which either prevent or immediately resolve thromboses as they occur.

Subsequent studies[32,33] have shown that stilbesterol dosages up to 3.0 mg/day do not cause the increased cardiovascular complications noted above, but will still depress the plasma testosterone to the castrate range. It is therefore advocated that stilbesterol in doses of 1.0 mg/day to 1.0 mg t.i.d. be used as initial therapy when hormonal treatment is begun.

V. OTHER ESTROGENS

A. Polyestradiol Phosphate

Polyestradiol phosphate (Estradurin®) is a polymer consisting of molecules of estradiol linked by phosphate bonds. When injected intramuscularly, the phosphate bonds are hydrolyzed sequentially, emitting a constant supply of estradiol. Treatment is by injection intramuscularly, 40 mg monthly. Estrogen treatment may be better tolerated in this manner and this medication appears as effective as stilbesterol.

B. Diethylstilbesterol Diphosphate (Stilphostrol®)

Diethylstilbesterol diphosphate is indicated when there has been failure of previously listed estrogens or of orchiectomy to control the manifestations of the disease. While this has the same tendency as other estrogens for adverse reactions, one can give Stilphostrol® intravenously at high dosages for a short period of time and achieve some measure of relief, particularly of ureteral obstruction or of bone pain, when this was not obtained on other estrogens at lower dosage. Stilphostrol® 0.5 g in 300 mℓ of saline or 5% dextrose is given intravenously for 1 or 2 days; each day thereafter, 1g is similarily administered for 5 days or more, depending on the response of the patient. The infusion should be adjusted so that the entire amount is given in a period of 1 hr.

C. Estracyt

This chemical combination of a nitrogen mustard and estradiol given intravenously has been reported by Lindberg[34] and Fossa and Miller[35] and found to be effective in advanced prostatic cancer, particularly in patients who have escaped or been refractory to other estrogens. The average durations of response was about 1 year. Mittelman et al.[36] have described oral administration. Favorable responses in the order of 20 to 40% have been reported by the National Prostatic Cancer project.[37] At present, the numbers of patients tested are small and the results thus far must be regarded as tentative. The compound has not been released by the U.S. Food and Drug Administration for general clinical usage.

VI. ORCHIECTOMY

A. Technique

Most urologists prefer bilateral epididymo-orchiectomy through an anterior transverse incision, allowing access successively into each of the scrotal compartments. Removal of both the testis and epididymis removes all known sources of testicular androgen. Some authors have favored removal of only the testis on each side, leaving the epididymis intact to remain as a cosmetic testis-like lump of tissue. Others have favored an intra-capsular parenchymectomy, leaving the capsule of the testis to be closed around a piece of fat or hemostatic foreign substance to more fully sustain the illusion that the testis is still present. Finally, testicular prostheses of life-like consistency are available for implantation.

About 90% of patients will show striking evidence of objective and subjective benefit, as shown by decrease in the size of the primary prostatic cancer, decrease or relief of bone pain, and decrease in the size of metastatic deposit and in the serum acid phosphatase. Other subjective improvements include increase in appetite and weight, a sense of euphoria, improvement in hematologic parameters, and rather striking change to a fairly normal lifestyle. Unfortunately, about 80% of those so benefited will show a relapse and return to their symptoms in approximately 1 year. Since there are no hormone changes such as increase in the serum testosterone, serum estrogens, or a change in ratio of these hormones to suggest a cause for relapse, we have been inclined to postulate that tumor cells have lost their dependence on androgenic stimulus and are now autonomous. More recently, Prout[38] has suggested that perhaps the androgen-sensitive cells have indeed been eradicated by the hormonal measures, but clones of cells which were never androgen dependent survive and gradually dominate the picture.

Most authors agree that stilbesterol in amounts of up to 3 mg/day is as effective as orchiectomy in bringing about the remission of symptoms of disseminated prostatic cancer. A controversy exists as to which entity should be employed first.

Stilbesterol doses of 1 mg/day will bring about relief of symptoms in many patients. Some of these patients will retain potency on this low dose of estrogen, which has been shown to lower serum testosterone but not to castrate levels. The disparity between estrogen effect and lowering of serum testosterone has been mentioned previously. After estrogens have been used and when relapse occurs, there is still a fairly considerable group of patients, up to 30% as recently reported by Gray and Bjorn,[39] who will get additional benefit from bilateral orchiectomy. These again will show subjective and objective improvement, as noticed in the first period of treatment with estrogens. For this reason, although some authors feel that these two entities are interchangeable, we believe that the period of beneficial suppression of prostatic cancer symptoms can be lengthened by employing estrogens first, starting with a dosage of 1 mg/day and ultimately increasing to 3 mg, followed by orchiectomy when required. In contrast, estrogen therapy after relapse from control by orchiectomy is seldom beneficial.

B. Adrenalectomy

The escape of patients from hormonal control following estrogen administration or orchiectomy prompted investigators to seek to control or ablate other sources of androgens. The adrenals came under consideration almost immediately.[40] Successful bilateral adrenalectomy awaited the advent of cortisone and the description of an operative protocol with management by cortisone administration for successful bilateral adrenalectomy in humans.[41] Although early reports were enthusiastic,[42-44] it was soon found that the duration of objective responses was too short to be of practical value to the patient and that this could be brought about by medical adrenalectomy. This attitude has persisted to the present time in the minds of most urologists. Exceptions are reports by Mahoney and Harris[45] and by the Roswell Park group,[46] in which they have described more significant and long-lasting benefits from adrenalectomy.

C. Hypophysectomy

The relative lack of success following bilateral adrenalectomy led investigators logically to consider hypophysectomy as the final step in ablative endocrine therapy. Most patients represent failures from estrogen and orchiectomy as attempts at control. As one reviews the list of reports (Table 1)[47] of hypophysectomy for prostatic cancer, one is impressed that the numbers of patients are small, ranging from 10 to 34, with the exception of Ferguson's evaluation of 100 patients, and that the mean duration of remission and mean survivals were short. Most attempts have either ended in disillusionment or a very rigid selection of patients for hypophysectomy. Reports have fea-

TABLE 1

Endocrine Ablative Procedures for Treatment of Carcinoma of the Prostate

Procedure	Series	Number of patients	5 Years	Survival percentage		Comments
				Other		
Hypophysectomy	Luft[74]	10		Mean duration of remission — 9 months		50% subjective 3 died postoperatively
	Smith[113]	5				80% objective remission
	Ray[101]	16				37% subjective improvement
	Scott[108]	17 (2 initial treatments)		Mean survival — 8 months		50% objective remission
	Straffon[119]	13		Mean survival — 5 months		3 died postoperatively 75% subjective improvement
	Ferguson[40]	100				70% subjective improvement
	Morales[84]		23			74% subjective improvement
	Murphy[90]		34	Mean survival — 8 months		35% subjective improvement
	Maddy[77]	20		Mean duration of remission — 7 months		63% subjective improvement
	West[133]	27		Mean survival — 8 months		37% objective remission
	Welvaart[130]	14		Mean survival — 10 months		43% subjective improvement

Modified from Resnick, M. I., and Grayhack, J. T., *Urol. Clin. Am.,* 2, 141, 1975. (With permission.)

tured principally subjective improvement, which ranged from 37 to 75%. The chief indication has been for generalized bone pain, too widespread for local control by spot radiotherapy. Our own experience has convinced us that hypophysectomy is an end-of-the-road maneuver which has about a 60 to 70% chance of relieving bone pain for a short period of days to weeks.

D. Prolactin Inhibitors

The synergistic role of prolactin in its relationship to testosterone as they affect prostatic growth and function has been discussed in Volume II, Chapter 1. Studies[48] have shown significant levels of specific prolactin binding sites in some hyperplastic prostate glands, as well as in prostatic adenocarcinoma; the significance of prolactin and prolactin receptors in the etiology or treatment of prostatic cancer is uncertain. Attempts to correlate prolactin receptor densities to hormonal responses in the prostate gland are in progress.

Prolactin-inhibiting compounds such as L-dopamine have recently been used[49] in patients with disseminated prostatic cancer, both to determine the effect of this treatment on pain and also possibly to predict the potential benefits of hypophysectomy.

Like hypophysectomy, the most marked effect has been in a nonspecific relief of pain, the nature of the subjective response being about 55%.

E. Antiandrogens

Antiandrogens are compounds which compete with dihydrotestosterone for intra-cellular androgen receptor sites and thus prevent the action of potent androgens on the prostatic target cell. The first of these compounds, cyproterone acetate, very similar to structure to testosterone, was examined extensively in a clinical trial sponsored by Shering Laboratories over the period 1965 to 1970. In this study, patients with disseminated prostatic cancer, either untreated or at least 1 month following cessation of other hormone treatment and without radiation treatment, were compared to the results produced by stilbesterol, 5 mg daily. The data accumulated from these studies showed that there was no essential advantage in cyproterone acetate over stilbesterol and the use of cyproterone acetate was not approved by the U.S. Food and Drug Administration for use in the U.S. A more potent antiandrogen, flutamide, has been studied more recently,[50] but the results have not been good enough to favor replacement of estrogens in the routine treatment of metastatic prostatic cancer. In addition, there seemed to be little effect in most cases when antiandrogens were employed after other hormonal means, particularly orchiectomy and estrogens, had failed.

F. Androgen Stimulation Followed by Radioactive Phosphorus

Occasionally, there is some benefit in a patient suffering severe generalized pain from disseminated prostatic cancer to stimulation of the cancer deposits with testosterone, followed by the administration of radioactive phosphorus. The androgen stimulation has now generally been replaced by parathormone administration, which also stimulates actively growing metastases to take up the phosphorus more avidly than normal tissues; the local irradiation may temporarily ameliorate pain. The benefits of such therapy are usually short lived, often less than a month.

VII. SUMMARY

In summary, the endocrinologic treatments of disseminated prostatic cancer rests on the use of estrogens, usually stilbesterol, as the first line of attack. After estrogen relapse has occurred, bilateral orchiectomy may again bring about objective and subjective remission in up to 30% of patients. Estracyt may be used as a substitute for stilbesterol or following escape from either of the above methods of hormonal control with an expectation of moderate response. The benefits of bilateral adrenalectomy, medical adrenalectomy by cortico-steroids, hypophysectomy, and prolactin-inhibiting agents tend to be nonspecific and of short duration.

REFERENCES

1. American Cancer Society: Cancer statistics, 1977, *Ca-A Cancer J. Clinicians,* 27, 1977.
2. **Whitmore, W. F., Jr.,** The rationale and result of abblative surgery for prostatic cancer, *Cancer (Philadelphia),* 16, 1119, 1963.
3. **Flocks, R. H., O'Donoghue, E. P., Millerman, L. A., and Culp, D. A.,** Management of stage C prostatic carcinoma, *Urol. Clin. North Am.,* 2, 163, 1975.
4. **Langstaff, G.,** Cases of fungus haematodes, *Medico-Chirurgical, Trans., London,* Vol. 8, part I, 279, 1817. (This later became the Royal Med. Chir. Soc. Trans.)

5. **Thompson, H.**, *The Enlarged Prostate, Its Pathology and Treatment,* John Churchill, London, 1858, 212.

6. **White, J. W.**, The results of double castration in hypertrophy of the prostate, *Ann Surg.,* 22, 1, 1895.

7. **Cabot, A. T.**, The question of castration for enlarged prostate, *Ann. Surg.,* 24, 265, 1896.

8. **Huggins, C., Masina, M. H., Eichelberger, L., and Wharton, J. D.**, Quantitative studies of prostatic secretion. I. Characteristics of the normal secretion: the influence of thyroid, suprarenal, and testis extirpation and androgen substitution on the prostatic output, *J. Exp. Med.,* 70, 543, 1939.

9. **Huggins, C. and Clark, P. J.**, Quantitative studies of prostatic secretion. II. The effect of castration and of estrogen injection of the normal and of the hyperplastic prostate gland of dogs, *J. Exp. Med.,* 72, 747, 1940.

10. **Kutscher, W. and Wolberg, H.**, Prostatphosphatase, *Z. Physiol. Chem.,* 236, 237, 1935.

11. **Gutman, A. B. and Gutman, E. G.**, An "acid" phosphatase occurring in the serum of patients with metastasizing carcinoma of the prostate gland, *J. Clin. Invest.,* 17, 473, 1938.

12. **Huggins, C. and Hodges, C. V.**, Studies of prostatic cancer. I. The effect of castration, of estrogen and of androgen injection on serum phosphatase in metastatic carcinoma of the prostate, *Cancer Res.,* 1, 293, 1941.

13. **Huggins, C., Stevens, R., and Hodges, C. V.**, Studies on prostatic cancer II. The effects of castration on advanced carcinoma of the prostate gland, *Arch. Surg.,* 43, 209, 1941.

14. **Hodges, C. V., Pearse, H. D., and Stille, L.**, Radical prostatectomy for carcinoma — 30 year experience and 15 year survivals, *J. Urol.,* in press.

15. **Cooper, J. F. and Foti, A.**, A radio immunoassay for prostatic acid phosphatase, I. Methodology and range of normal male serum values, *Invest. Urol.,* 12, 98, 1974.

16. **Wajsman, Z., Chu, T. M., Saroff, J., and Murphy, G. P.**, A National Field Trial of Two New, Direct and Specific Acid Phosphatase Determination, Material presented at annual American Urological Association, Inc. meeting, Washington, D. C., May, 1978.

17. **Veeneman, R. J., Gursel, E. O., Romas, N., Wechsler, M., and Lattimer, J. K.**, Bone marrow acid phosphatase: prognostic value in patients undergoing radical prostatectomy, *J. Urol.,* 117, 81, 1977.

18. **Pontes, J. E., Choe, B. K., Rose, N. R., and Pierce, J. M., Jr.**, Bone marrow acid phosphatase in staging of prostatic cancer; how reliable is it?, *J. Urol.,* 119, 772, 1978.

19. **McCullough, D. L., McLaughlin, A. E., III, and Gittes, R. F.**, Morbidity of pelvic lymphadenectomy and radical prostatectomy for prostatic cancer, *J. Urol.,* 117, 206, 1977.

20. Veterans Administration Co-operative Urological Research Group (VACURG). Treatment and survival of patients with cancer of the prostate, *Surg. Gynecol. Obstet.,* 124, 1011, 1967.

21. **Resnick, M. I. and Grayhack, J. T.**, Treatment of stage IV carcinoma of the prostate, *Urol. Clin. North Am.,* 2, 141, 1975.

22. **Baird, D. T., Uno, A., and Melby, J. C.**, Adrenal secretion of androgens and estrogens, *J. Endocrinology,* 45, 135, 1969.

23. **Flocks, R. H., Marberger, H., Begley, B. J., and Prendergast, L. J.**, Prostatic carcinoma, treatment of advance cases with intravenous diethylstilbestrol diphosphate, *J. Urol.,* 74, 549, 1955.

24. **Goodwin, D. W., Rasmussen-Taxdal, D. S., Ferreira, A. A., and Scott, W. W.**, Estrogen inhibition of androgen-maintained prostatic secretion in the hpophysectomized dog, *J. Urol.,* 86, 134, 1961.

26. **Young, H. H., II. and Kent, J. R.**, Plasma testosterone levels in patients with prostatic carcinoma before and after treatment, *J. Urol.,* 99, 788, 1968.

27. **Robinson, M. R. G. and Thomas, D. S.**, Effect of hormonal therapy on plasma testosterone levels in prostatic carcinoma, *Br. Med. J.,* 4, 391, 1971.

28. **Mackler, M. A., Liberti, J. P., Smith, M. J. V., et al.**, The effect of orchiectomy and various doses of stilbesterol on plasma testosterone levels in patients with carcinoma of the prostate, *Invest. Urol.,* 9, 423, 1972.

29. **Kent, J. R., Bischoft, A. J., Ardyno, L. J., et al.**, Estrogen dosage and suppression of testosterone levels in patients with prostatic carcinoma, *J. Urol.,* 109, 858, 1973.

30. **Shearer, R. J., Hendry, W. F., Sommerville, I. F., et al.**, Plasma testosterone: an accurate monitor of hormone treatment in prostatic cancer, *Br. J. Urol.,* 45, 668, 1973.

31. **Baker, H. W. G., Burger, H. G., DeKretser, D. M., et al.**, Effects of synthetic oral oestrogens in normal men and patients with prostatic carcinoma: lack of gonadotrophin suppression by chlorotrianisene, *Clin. Endocrinol.,* 2, 297, 1973.

32. **Byer, D. P.**, The Veterans Administration Co-Operative Urologic Research Group's studies of cancer of the prostate, *Cancer (Philadelphia),* 32, 1126, 1973.

33. **Blackard, C. E.**, The Veterans Administration Co-Operative Urologic Research Group's studies of carcinoma of the prostate: a review, *Cancer Chemother. Rep.,* 59, 225, 1975.

34. **Lindberg, B.,** Treatment of rapidly progressing prostatic carcinoma with Estracyt, *J. Urol.,* 108, 303, 1972.
35. **Fossa, S. D. and Miller, A.,** Treatment of advanced carcinoma of the prostate with estramustine phosphate, *J. Urol.,* 115, 406, 1976.
36. **Mittelman, A. P., Shukla, S. K., and Murphy, G. P.,** Extended therapy of stage D carcinoma of the prostate with oral estramustine phosphate, *J. Urol.,* 115, 409, 1976.
37. **Murphy, G. P.,** Management of advanced cancer of the prostate, *Genito-Urinary Cancer,* Skinner, D. G. and DeKernion, J. B., Eds., W. B. Saunders, 1978, chap. 22.
38. **Prout, G. R., Jr.,** Prostate gland, *Cancer Medicine,* Vol. 25(4), Holland, James F., and Frei, Emil, III, Eds., Lea & Febiger, Philadelphia, 1973.
39. **Bjorn, C. L., Gray, C. P., and Strauss, E.,** Orchiectomy after Presumed Estrogen Failure in Treatment of Carcinoma of the Prostate, presented at Annual Meeting of Western Section, American Urological Association, Seattle, Washington, July, 1978.
40. **Huggins, C. B. and Scott, W. W.,** Bilateral adrenalectomy in prostatic cancer. Clinical features and urinary excretion of 17-Ketosteroids and estrogen, *Ann. Surg.,* 122, 1031, 1945.
41. **Huggins, C. B. and Bergenstal, D.,** Inhibition of human mammary and prostatic cancers by adrenalectomy, *Cancer Res.,* 12, 134, 1952.
42. **Baker, W. J.,** Bilateral adrenalectomy for carcinoma of the prostate gland; preliminary report, *J. Urol.,* 70, 275, 1953.
43. **Whitmore, W. F., Randall, H. T., Pearson, O. H., and West, C. D.,** Adrenalectomy in the treatment of prostatic cancer, *Geriatrics,* 9, 62, 1954.
44. **Morales, P. A., Brendler, H., and Hotchkiss, R. S.,** The role of the adrenal cortex on prostatic cancer, *J. Urol.,* 73, 399, 1955.
45. **Mahoney, E. M. and Harrison, J. H.,** Bilateral adrenalectomy for palliative treatment of prostatic cancer, *J. Urol.,* 108, 936, 1972.
46. **Bhanalaph, T., Varkarakis, M. J., and Murphy, G. P.,** Current status of bilateral adrenalectomy for advanced prostatic carcinoma, *Am. Surg.,* 179, 17, 1974.
47. **Resnick, M. I. and Grayhack, J. T.,** Treatment of stage IV prostatic carcinoma, *Urol. Clin. North Am.,* 2, 141, 1975.
48. **Keenan, E. J., Kemp, E. D., Ramsey, E. E., Garrison, L. B., Pearse, H. D., and Hodges, C. V.,** Specific binding of prolactin by the prostate gland of the rat and man, *J. Urol.,* in press, 1978.
49. **Farnsworth, W. E. and Gonder, M. J.,** Prolactin and prostate cancer, *Urology,* 10, 33, 1977.
50. **Stolear, B. and Albert, D. J.,** SCH — 13521 in the treatment of advanced carcinoma of the prostate, *J. Urol.,* 111, 803, 1974.

Chapter 3

HORMONAL THERAPY OF RENAL-CELL CARCINOMA

Thomas F. Hogan*

TABLE OF CONTENTS

*   This work was supported by NIH-NCI Grant T32-CA 09075. Dr. Hogan is a Clinical Fellow of the American Cancer Society.

I. INTRODUCTION

A. Clinical Problem

Renal-cell carcinoma (RCC) or hypernephroma accounts for 80% of all renal malignancies and occurs in about 9100 persons per year in the U.S. The disease is found twice as often in men,[1] and the incidence increases steadily after age 30, with an average age of onset of 61 years for men and 63 years for women. There has been a slowly increasing, age-adjusted incidence rate in men, which somewhat parallels that of pancreatic carcinoma.[2] Unfortunately, the extent of the disease at the time of diagnosis has remained static for the past decade, and about half of all patients present with locally advanced (Stage 3) or metastatic (Stage 4) disease. The 5-year survival in these cases is usually 10% or less.[1,2]

B. Past Rationale for Hormonal Therapy

The kidney is a known target organ for a variety of hormones, including antidiuretic hormone, aldosterone, and parathormone. In addition, androgens cause renal hypertrophy in rats and mice, and estrogens induce renal malignancy in hamsters.[3] A circadian mitotic rhythm occurs in both frog proximal convoluted tubule and frog renal carcinoma tissue.[4] Both normal kidney and RCC tissue may synthesize various hormones. Although polycythemia occurs in only 2 to 10% of patients with RCC,[5-7] Sufrin et al.[8] found elevated plasma erythropoietin (ESF) levels in 63% of 57 patients studied. Murphy et al.[6] assayed ESF, using the rate of incorporation of ^{59}Fe into the erythrocytes of adult mice. He found elevated levels in RCC patients with localized tumors. These elevated plasma ESF levels decreased to normal after nephrectomy, but persisted after nephrectomy in patients with metastatic disease, suggesting that the residual RCC tissue was the hormone source. Furthermore, Sherwood and Goldwasser[9] directly identified ESF in the cell-culture media from both clear-cell and granular-cell explants of human RCC. Although Sufrin et al.[8] found elevated plasma renin concentrations in 37% of their 57 RCC patients, it is not yet known whether this hormone is produced directly by the malignant tissue. Similar reports regarding chorionic gonadotropin[5,8,10] also lack the demonstration of ectopic hormone secretion by RCC tissue.

The above evidence for a hormonal influence on renal tissue is supported by the epidemiology of human RCC. These tumors are uncommon during childhood, and, when they do occur, the incidence in males is equal to that in females.[11] In adults, however, the incidence of both renal cortical adenomas, which are probably premalignant lesions, and RCC is higher in men than women, as is the reported frequency of spontaneous disease regression.[3,12-14] Noting these trends, Bloom first demonstrated that hormonal manipulation inhibited tumor induction and growth in the stilbestrol-induced hamster renal carcinoma.[15,16] He then proceeded to apply hormonal therapy to human RCC.

Much of the subsequent impetus for hormonal manipulation in the treatment of advanced RCC has come from Bloom's work.[3,12,15-20] He began treating RCC patients with androgens and progestogens in the 1960s. In 1973, the results from 80 patients were reported; 11 were described as showing an objective response and 2 had "stable disease", giving an overall response rate of 16%.[13] Although Van der Werf-Messing and Van Gilse[21] questioned the use of pulmonary metastases for gauging clinical response in RCC, many clinicians accepted Bloom's report and in 1973, he listed eight other series where progestogens and/or androgens were used in the treatment of these tumors. Seven of these series appeared to confirm the original findings.[13]

C. Current Questions

The published results of early clinical trials have encouraged the widespread use of hormones in the treatment of advanced RCC. A review of the case records of 129 patients with RCC, seen at the University of Wisconsin between 1969 and 1975, revealed that 55 were treated with progestogens and 34 with androgens, both for an average treatment duration of 3 months. In addition, 23 patients received glucocorticoid or estrogen therapy for short intervals. Because the average time from tissue diagnosis to death for patients presenting with metastatic disease was approximately 14 months, and progestogens and androgens were always used sequentially, it follows that hormonal therapy occupied a major part of these patients' survival period.[22] It becomes important, therefore, to determine whether confirmatory clinical or laboratory data have evolved since 1963 which confirm the benefit of hormonal therapy for RCC.

II. ANDROGENS IN RENAL-CELL CARCINOMA

A. Metabolic Studies

There are limited data on androgen metabolism in patients with RCC. Böttinger and Lisboa[23] analyzed urine samples from 15 patients, and found normal total daily urinary 17-ketosteroid excretion and etiocholanolone to androsterone ratios. Bojar et al.[24] incubated preparations of normal renal tubules from seven male RCC patients with ^{14}C-labeled testosterone. They found that, with time, an increasing amount of the radioactivity was recovered as unidentified androgen metabolites. Thus, normal human kidney did contribute to the extrahepatic metabolism of testosterone. Similar studies were not performed on the adjacent RCC tissue.

The microsomes, endoplasmic reticulum and nuclei of androgen target tissues, such as prostate, contain a reductase which converts testosterone (T) to dihydrotestosterone (DHT).[25-27] Both DHT and T bind to specific androphilic proteins. A DHT/T ratio of 3:1 was found in both prostatic cytosol and nuclei prepared from hepatectomized, male rats, indicating that DHT is more avidly bound to the receptor than T.[28] The reduction of T to yield DHT is competitively inhibited by the progestogen gestonorone,[29] and also by high levels of estrogens or progesterone.[27,29]

Unlike prostate, normal kidney contains little testosterone reductase activity;[27] oxidation to androstenedione and epitestosterone appear to be the major renal metabolic fates of T in man. Marberger et al.[29] used ^{3}H-testosterone to examine androgen metabolism in vitro by renal tissue slices. Normal kidney oxidized 61%, and RCC 22%, of the added ^{3}H-testosterone to androstenedione and epitestosterone. The progestational antiandrogen gestonorone, which only inhibits T reduction, had little effect on androgen metabolism by these tissues. It was concluded from these data that gestonorone was unlikely to be therapeutically effective against the human RCC. However, as tissues from only six RCC specimens were examined, further work with gestonorone and other antiandrogens may be warranted.

B. Receptor Proteins

Both normal and malignant tissues may contain androgen-receptor proteins.[26,27,30] However, work with testicular feminization models[27,31] showed that neither androgen uptake nor measurable androgen-receptor content provide conclusive proof that there is a significant androgenic effect on the tissue in question. Androgen-receptor content may vary with age,[27] the degree of sexual maturation,[32] and tissue exposure to other hormones.[33] Also, differing androgenic effects may occur in receptor-containing tissues; for example, DNA synthesis predominates in prostate, whereas RNA and protein synthesis predominate in kidney.[34]

Fanestil et al.[35] assayed androgen binding by five human RCC specimens and corresponding normal tissues. Slices were incubated with ³H-T, the cytosol and nuclear fractions separated, and displacement analysis performed by the addition of a 100-fold excess of unlabeled T. The binding of T to the nuclei was 15 times greater in the malignant tissue, and cytosol binding was two to three-fold greater. This assay, however, did not take account of nonspecific binding and does not prove conclusively that specific androgen receptors are present in RCC. There do not appear to be any other publications in which RCC tissue was assayed for androgen receptor content.

C. Laboratory Models

Androgens enhance the growth of rat and mouse kidney,[32,36,37] and, although there is no direct trophic effect on hamster kidney, some androgen-induced renal enzyme changes do occur in this species.[38] Whether or not exogenous androgens induce cancers in laboratory animals is still unsettled.[39,40] A promotional effect of androgenic steroids on chemical carcinogenesis has been demonstrated in mice but not rats. Noronha[37] gave intraperitoneal injections of dimethylnitrosamine (DMN) to inbred NZO/Black mice, a strain which normally has an 0.3% incidence of spontaneous renal malignancy. When 15 mg/kg of DMN was administered to 21 female mice and 20 castrated males, none developed renal tumors. However, 12 of 21 intact males did develop renal tumors. Weisburger et al.[41] reported that the renal-tubule carcinogen, streptozotocin, at a dose of 6 to 12 mg/kg, induced renal tumors in 18 of 30 male mice (60%), but in only 7 of 39 females (18%).[40] It is not known whether this tumor enhancement occurred via a direct or indirect androgen effect on the kidney. In contrast to mice, similar experiments with rats did not demonstrate any androgenic stimulation of tumor production or growth.[41,42]

A report by Kauffman[43] found is little direct androgenic effect on human RCC suspensions transferred to the cheek pouches of hamsters pretreated with cortisone. RCC xenografts grew reproducibly, could be serially transplanted, and had measurable growth inhibition when various chemotherapeutic agents were used. However, both testosterone and a placebo produced growth inhibition in only 1 of 80 grafts. Experimental details, such as testosterone dosage, frequency and duration of treatment, and the time of tumor measurement were not given. Other reports, dealing with the organ culture of human RCC explants, did not observe unequivocal histological changes when androgens were added to the medium.[44,45]

Autoradiographic studies on human RCC slices are of interest. Liao and coworkers[26,27] applied this technique to mice, and found that ³H-labeled T was retained in target tissues for 6 to 16 hr, but cleared from nontarget tissue after 1 hr. The parenchymal cells of target tissues took up the tracer avidly, but there was only a sparse accumulation in surrounding smooth muscle cells, and none by connective tissue. The label was present in nuclear chromatin from 0.5 to 7 hr after administration, but did not bind to nucleoli, even though androgens are known to enhance nucleolar RNA polymerase activity.[26,27] Studies of this sort might identify not only specific binding of androgens by human RCC, but also which cell type is involved: normal tubule cells, stromal cells, or malignant "clear" or "granular" cells.

D. Clinical Results

Although epidemiologic data, metabolic studies, experience with animal models, and androgen-receptor assays all suggest a possible relationship between androgens and human RCC, the results of therapeutic trials are best described as "dismal". Table 1 summarizes data from 13 studies performed since 1967; the overall objective response rate in a total of 232 patients was approximately 4%.

TABLE 1

Androgen Clinical Trials in Renal-Cell Carcinoma

Date	Agent	Dose (mg)	Average Duration	Objective Responses	Comment	Ref.
1967	TP	140, 2×/week	3 months	1/15	Partial response	46
1968	T	100/day	6 weeks	1/11	Partial response	47
1969	A	100—300/week	—	0/11	Given after progestogens	14
1969	TP	100/day	4 weeks	3/9	Partial response	48
1970	T	—	—	0/6	—	49
1971	TP or TC	100/day × 5 400/week	—	2/27	One partial response was 25% decrease in tumor diameter for 30 days; also, one complete response	50
1971	TP	50, 3×/week	—	0/2	—	21
1973	F or T or TCP	30/day 100, 3×/week 200/week	—	0/37	27 men, 10 women	51
1974	TP/TR	200/week × 3	—	0/23	—	52
1975	FM	20/day	8—12 weeks	1/20	Partial response, 20% decrease in tumor diameter; no increase in survival notes	53
1975	T	300/week	—	0/37	—	54
1977	TP	500/week	—	1/16	Partial response, four others are excluded (see text)	55
1978	F	10—40/day	3 months	0/5	"Response" was 50% decrease of all measurable lesions	22
	TL	200/week	3 months	0/1		
	TP	400—600/week	3 months	0/5		
	TE	200—600/week	3 months	0/7		
Grand Total:				9/232	Total responses, 1 complete and 8 partial, equals 4%	

Note: A, unspecified androgens; F, Fluoxymesterone, oral; T, testosterone, intramuscular; TC, testosterone cypionate, intramuscular; TCP, testosterone cyclopentyl propionate, intramuscular; TE, testosterone enanthate, intramuscular; TP, testosterone propionate, intramuscular; TL, testolactone; TR, triandrolone.

Ideally, the term "objective response" should be so defined that reports from different institutions can be compared with confidence. The definition of response is critical when hormonal therapies are being evaluted, because these agents may give subjective improvement without having any true antitumor effect, and without influencing survival. Many oncologic groups now use rigorous "partial response" criteria, which are similar to those proposed by the National Cancer Institute for breast carcinoma. These require a 50% or more decrease in the sum of the size of all tumor masses, with no more than a 25% increase in any single lesion, which lasts for at least 4 weeks. Such responses usually mean that disease palliation and prolonged survival are achieved, and these criteria make possible the comparison of results from different institutions.

The reports of androgen responses given in Table 1 generally employed less rigorous criteria than those which are currently accepted, and did not document whether or not there had been an improvement in patient survival. For example, even in a recent report[55] which claimed five responses to hormones in 20 patients, only one tumor response met the above criteria. The other four responses included a previously irradiated bone lesion, a patient with stable hepatic involvement, and two patients in whom the response was described as only "minimal in extent".

E. Summary

Normal human kidney can metabolize androgens, but the pathways may differ from those of classic target tissues such as the prostate. Studies on androgen metabolism in RCC tissue slices are indicated, because they may reveal pathways which are essential to tumor growth and amenable to blockade by antiandrogens.

Androgen-receptor assays on RCC tissue may be difficult to correlate with the results of therapy, because so few patients, less than 5% in the series cited, respond to androgens. Also, there are many variables which could affect assay results. These include the techniques used, the influence of other hormones on receptor content, the age and metabolic status of the patient, ligand metabolism occurring during the assay, receptors being present but having affinity for androgens other than the ones being used as probes, and the fact that tissues exist which contain androgen receptors, but which are exempt from androgen effects. In any event, to-date there has been no major attempt to measure androgen receptor proteins in human RCC tissue, and one cannot exclude the possibility that a subset of patients may have androgen- or antiandrogen-influenced tumors.

Yet, although there are tantalizing hints that androgens are somehow involved in renal metabolism and growth, they cannot be recommended as standard therapy for human RCC at the present time. They may be indicated, however, as a palliative measure; for example, in the treatment of anemia and anorexia. Further clinical — endocrinologic research may yet define a role for "androgen manipulation" in RCC.

III. PROGESTOGENS IN RENAL-CELL CARCINOMA

A. General Comments

Progestogens are mildly catabolic in man. This effect is dose dependent, with 50 mg of progesterone per day increasing urinary nitrogen excretion and decreasing plasma amino acid levels.[47] The synthetic progestogen medroxyprogesterone acetate (MPA), at a dose of 25 to 50 mg daily does not affect nitrogen balance, but higher doses do inhibit the anabolic effects of testosterone and fluoxymesterone.[56] MPA affects pituitary—adrenal function.[57] It causes a reduction in the plasma growth hormone response to insulin stimulation and arginine infusion,[47] and decreases gonadotropin production with a resulting loss of libido.[20,47,56,58] In one endocrine study,[59] RCC patients treated with 600 mg of MPA per week were found to have reduced plasma LH concentrations, and all of five males had low plasma T concentrations. Plasma TSH levels were unchanged. Although the effect on urinary estrogen excretion was variable, 7 of the 16 patients had definitely reduced levels.

Early reports described MPA as having only low glucocorticoid potency.[18,56,58] However, doses recommended by Bloom[18] for the treatment of RCC (300 to 400 mg per day) produce significant glucocorticoid effects,[47] and patients may experience steroid euphoria.[56] MPA can be substituted for cortisol to prevent canine renal allograft rejection.[20,57] Sadoff and Lusk[59] noted decreased plasma cortisol levels in 11 of 16 RCC patients who received 600 mg of MPA per week for 8 weeks; five were tested with metyrapone and all showed blunted ACTH responses. None of these 16 patients developed clinical evidence of glucocorticoid deficiency while receiving MPA. Hellman et al.[57] also observed low plasma cortisol levels, reduced cortisol production rates, and blunted responses to exogenous ACTH in MPA-treated patients.

These observations on MPA's glucocorticoid effects are important to the present discussion, because MPA has been recommended for the treatment of RCC.[3,12,15,16,18-20] There do not appear to be any published reports of progesterone metabolic studies in patients with RCC, or attempts to alter RCC growth by manipulating progesterone metabolic pathways.

B. Receptor Proteins

Faber et al.[60] have reviewed the estrogen-induced biosynthesis, structure, and nuclear binding of mammalian progesterone receptor proteins (PR). These proteins can be isolated on sucrose density gradients, but the progesterone affinity constant may vary by 100%, depending on the buffers used and the isolation conditions.

Pasqualini et al.[61] employed a sucrose gradient technique to measure hormone receptors in fetal guinea pig kidney at 35 to 55 days gestation. Although aldosterone and estrogen receptors were demonstrated, PR was not present at this stage of development. Few attempts to assay PR in human kidney have been reported. Fanestil et al.[35] incubated thin slices of human kidney and adjacent RCC tissue with 6×10^{-9} M ^{3}H-labeled progesterone. Cytosol and nuclei were obtained, and the amount of radioactivity displaced by a 100-fold excess of unlabeled steroid was measured. Four patient-samples were studied; the normal and tumor nuclei bound 1.70 ± 0.86 and 18.7 ± 12.6 fmol progesterone per milligram protein, respectively. It was concluded that some human renal tumors may be susceptible to steroidal regulation. Concolino et al.[62] reported agar gel electrophoresis data from three human kidneys removed for renal lithiasis. Cytosol was first incubated with cortisol to saturate corticosteroid-binding globulin, then with dextran-charcoal to remove endogenous free steroids, and, finally, with ^{3}H-labeled progesterone. Electrophoresis demonstrated the presence of specific PR in these three samples, quantitation in two giving values of 11 and 39 fmol progesterone per milligram protein. These workers subsequently studied 10 RCC; 9 contained PR, with more binding sites and higher binding capacity, but lower receptor affinity, than that found in the normal kidney.[63] Tumor differentiation did not correlate with binding capacity, and follow-up was too short to relate receptor status to clinical results in progestogen-treated patients.

C. Laboratory Models

Progestogens, like androgens, induce hypertrophy of rat and mouse kidney,[15] but progestogen-induced renal carcinomas have not been observed in either species. It is not known whether synergism occurs between progestogens and chemical carcinogens in experimental RCC induction.

The Kirkman stilbestrol-induced hamster renal carcinoma is inhibited by progestogens.[15] This model provided the rationale for applying progestational therapy to human RCC, because the tumor, which is discussed further in Section IV.C., was inhibited during both the stilbestrol induction phase and during a later "estrogen-independent" phase. Tumor suppression by progestogens is not, however, a universal property of estrogen-dependent renal carcinoma in animals. A shows a spontaneous Balb C/cr mouse RCC estrogen enhanced tumor growth, while progestogens do not slow tumor progression.

As with androgens, there is little evidence that human RCC tissue explants are inhibited by a direct antitumor effect when exposed to progestogens. Tchao et al.[44] succeeded in growing 6 of 13 human explants in vitro, and MPA appeared to limit growth in two of them. However, Card and co-workers[45] exposed eight tumors in vitro to supraphysiologic levels of progesterone, and noted histological changes suggestive of inhibition in only 1 of 14 fragments from the eight tumors. Human serum produced similar "inhibition" in two or five fragments. Kaufman[43] studied human RCC suspensions transplanted to hamster cheek pouches which had been pretreated with cortisone. Both MPA and a placebo inhibited growth in only 1 of the 80 explants, suggesting that there was no direct progestational effect in this model system.

D. Clinical Results

Table 2 summarizes 22 studies completed since 1967, in which progestogens were used to treat RCC in over 500 patients. Originally, Bloom[12] reported that between 1959 and 1965, he had treated 38 patients with advanced RCC, and that an objective improvement had occurred in one androgen-treated, and seven progestogen-treated patients. This series was expanded, and in 1971, he reported that 12 of 79 patients treated with MPA achieved objective responses.[18] Although 3 of the 80 cases were considered to have a steroid-induced acceleration of tumor growth, two while receiving a progestogen and one during androgen therapy, the survival of the responders averaged 19.6 months, compared with 5.2 months for the nonresponders.

Although the survival difference was considered to demonstrate the efficacy of progestogen therapy, this study fails to meet present-day standards for cancer therapeutic trials. Tumor response criteria were not as rigorous as those in current use, and 4 of the 12 "responders" should probably be called "mixed" responses (Table 3). Even if the remaining eight cases do meet current criteria for an objective response, the actual tumor response rate for this study is only 10%. Also, it is possible that patients with less aggressive cancers, who had prolonged periods of stable disease, were included among the progestogen responders. Their extended survival might then have been interpreted erroneously as indicating a positive hormonal effect. Similar problems arise when reviewing other reports where prolonged survival was claimed for patients "responding" to MPA.[47]

Several of the other studies listed in Table 2 applied insufficiently rigorous criteria, and it is questionable whether they can be accepted as establishing the efficacy of progestogen therapy. For example, the two regressions described by Talley et al.[14] were observed 5 and 8 months after treatment, which calls into question their relationship to the progestogen therapy. Paine et al.[49] reported three progestogen responses, but one patient had bone progression while a lung lesion diminished, and another, although showing reduction in a pleural effusion, exhibited progression of a lung mass. Clearly, these should be categorized as "mixed responses", and only one objective response from this study is listed in Table 2.

Wagle and Murphy[50] reported three "partial responses" to MPA, but the evaluating criterion only required a 25% reduction in tumor size. Unless these cases and their survival are compared to previous methods of treatment used at the same institution, it is difficult to conclude that any real palliation or increase in survival took place.

Talley[51] reported five complete and two "partial" responses of pulmonary metastases in 61 progestogen-treated patients. Although the partial responses represented only some decrease in the size of the measured lesions, and not a 50% reduction, the five complete responses are of considerable interest. They provide the strongest support, to date, in favor of progestogen therapy for RCC. Even so, the complete response rate would be only 8%. Also, no soft tissue or brain responses were reported.

Peterson et al.[70] observed three responses in 14 patients treated with a small dose of MPA, but only one meets current response criteria, and is included in Table 2. The two reports by Hahn,[71,72] on behalf of the Eastern Cooperative Oncology Group, applied strict 50% tumor-response criteria. The first was of a prospective, randomized trial with megestrol acetate as one treatment arm; no responses were noted. The second trial compared treatment with vinblastine or Semustine (methyl CCNU), and these

TABLE 2

Progestogen Clinical Trials in Renal-Cell Carcinoma

Date	Agent	Dose (mg)	Objective Responses	Comment	Ref.
1967	P	—	1/4	Partial response	65
1967	A/P	—	4/20	Partial response	66
1968	MPA	100/day or 400/week	3/22	Partial response, increased survival?	47
1969	HC	1000/week	1/8	Two partial responses	14
	MPA	800/week	1/8	after 5 and 8 months of therapy	
1969	MPA	900/day × 4—8 week	0/9		48
1970	MPA	300/day	1/15	Partial response, two others excluded (see text)	49
1971	MPA	300/day	8/79	Partial response, four others excluded as"mixed" (see Table 3); increased survival?	18
1971	NSC	300/day × 6 week	0/27	—	67
1971	MPA	800/week	6/37	Partial responses, 25% decrease in tumor	50
1971	M	60/day	1/13	Partial responses, one response termed "doubtful" by author	21
	NC	200, 3 ×/week	1/9		
	MPA	50/day	1/9		
1972	ED or M or MG	50—60/day	1/11	Partial response, but equivocal	68
1973	MPA	1000/week × 4, then 400/week	7/61	Two partial responses were any decrease in tumor size; other five were complete	51
1974	MPA	600/week × 4—8 week	0/3	—	59
1974	OC	100/day	0/17	MPA given alone or in combination	52
	MPA	—	0/20		
1974	MPA	400/week	2/19	Partial responses, 50% decrease in tumor size	69
1974	MPA	40/day	1/14	Partial responses, two others excluded (see text)	70
1975	P	—	0/23	—	54
1975	MPA	300/day × 8 week	0/18	—	53
1976	M	150/m²/day	0/11	—	71
1976	MPA	800/week	7/76	Partial responses; MPA given together with chemotherapy	72
1977	PRO	800/week	0/15	One response excluded (see text)	55
1978	M	160/day	0/17	Response criterion was 50% decrease in measurable disease	22
	HC	1500/week	0/5		
	MPA	500/week oral or 750/week i.m.	0/20		
Grand Total:	MPA		37/410 (9%)	Total responses: five complete with MPA, all others were partial	
	M		1/41 (2%)		
	All others		8/139 (6%)		

Note: A/P, unspecified androgen/progestogen combinations; ED, ethynodiol diacetate, oral; HC, hydroxyprogesterone caproate, i.m.; M, megestrol, oral; MG, melengestrol, oral; MPA, medroxyprogesterone acetate, oral or i.m.; NC, norprogesterone caproate, i.m.; NSC — 17256, an experimental progestogen; OC, oxyprogesterone caproate, i.m.; P, unspecified progestogens; PRO, progesterone, i.m.

TABLE 3

Four Patients from a Clinical Trial of Medroxyprogesterone Acetate[18] with Questionable Tumor Responses Using Present-Day Standards

Patient	Reported Response Criteria
1. BS, female, age 58	Renal tumor approximately one third original size, but liver unchanged; death 3 months after starting progestogen therapy
2. AP, male, age 70	Pulmonary metastases continued to regress; progressive destruction of the femoral stump required hip disarticulation
3. WD, male, age 59	Some regression of pulmonary metastasis; abdomen still distended by large liver and ascites; death at home 3 months after starting medroxyprogesterone
4. EG, male, age 58	Reduction of abdominal mass; lung deposit unchanged throughout

drugs were added with MPA in a weekly dose of 800 mg. The treatment arms with the hormonal therapy showed no increase in response rate, and had a slightly worse median survival time.

Papec et al.[55] reported recalcification of a bony lesion in one of 16 patients treated with progesterone. However, this patient had received prior bone irradiation, and was also given an androgen at the same time as the progestogen.

Hogan[22] employed as his response criterion a 50% decrease of all measurable lesions for a 1-month period, with no new lesions. No patient from a total of 42 treated with MPA, megestrol acetate, or hydroxyprogesterone caproate showed a response to progestogen therapy (Table 2).

When the response rates in Table 2 are totaled, ignoring response definitions except to exclude obvious "mixed" responses and "stable-disease" cases, the overall figures are 9% for MPA (37/410), 2% for megestrol acetate (1/41), and 6% for other progestogens (8/139).

E. Summary

The evaluation of clinical trials in which progestogens were used to treat RCC is complicated by the glucocorticoid-like effects, differences in the dosage schedules employed, the variation in response criteria, and the lack of careful survival analysis which is found in most reports. In the case of MPA, the glucocorticoid effect is important when reviewing the earlier trials, because subjective responses were sometimes emphasized as much as tumor measurements. We have reviewed 22 studies involving 590 evaluable patients who were treated with a variety of progestogens. Using the current cooperative, oncology-group, response criteria, the response rates in these clinical trials fall below the 10% level. Even if the primary criterion of success is disease stabilization and prolongation of survival, the progestogens appear of little value; no survival benefit was found in two Eastern Cooperative Oncology Group studies in which patients were randomized to treatment arms with or without progestogens.[71,72]

To date, biological studies also fail to support a role for progestational agents in the treatment of human RCC. Inhibition of the Kirkman renal carcinoma by progestogens appears to be unique; progestogens do not, for example, inhibit an estrogen-supported murine renal carcinoma model. Also, there is evidence against a direct antitumor effect of progestogens on human RCC tissue in vitro. On the other hand, little is known about progesterone metabolism in patients with RCC, and recent data suggest that these tumors contain progesterone-receptor proteins. Further work in this area may well define a subset of patients who would benefit from progestational therapy. Thus far, however, progestogens cannot be recommended as a standard therapy for human RCC, despite the plethora of poorly documented reports to the contrary.

IV. ESTROGENS AND RENAL-CELL CARCINOMA

A. General Comments

Pituitary follicle-stimulating hormone (FSH) induces ovarian production of estradiol (E_2), estrone (E_1), and estriol (E_3). The 24-hr urinary-estriol excretion quotient, defined as the ratio of E_3 to $E_1 + E_2$, reflects the 16α-hydroxylation of E_1 and E_2, with population subgroups representing high, intermediate, and low levels of 16α-hydroxylation. It has been postulated that approximately 50% of Caucasian and 10% of other racial groups have inherited hydroxylation defects that are responsible for low, estriol-excretion quotients.[36] There are no reports describing the estriol-excretion quotients of RCC patients, but recent epidemiologic studies relate the incidence of this tumor in women to obesity, animal-fat consumption, and other factors which have been implicated in the hormonal etiology of carcinoma of the breast and endometrium[73] (see Chapters 2 and 4). In view of these data, investigations of estrogen metabolism in RCC patients may prove of considerable interest.

B. Receptor Proteins

Specific estrogen receptors (ER) are present in uterus, vagina, breast, prostate, epididymis, testis, liver, hypothalamus, pituitary, and kidney.[27,74] The occurrence of ER in a tissue implies that it is responsive to estrogen stimulation, and also that the estrogen is capable of inducing the synthesis of progesterone-receptor protein.[36,62]

Several recent reports have dealt with ER assays in mammalian kidney. De Vries et al.[76] administered 40 μg of estradiol per day to adrenalectomized Wistar-Lewis rats, and, using chromatographic techniques, determined that up to 54 fmol of the estrogen was bound per milligram of renal cytosol protein. Pasqualini et al.[61] used a sucrose-density gradient technique to study steroid binding by fetal guinea pig kidney at 35 to 55 days of gestation. Both renal-cell nuclei and cytosol contained distinct, specific estradiol and aldosterone-receptor proteins, with no competition by androgens or cortisol. ER assays have also been performed on human RCC.

Bojar et al.[77] studied tumor tissue from six untreated men with nonmetastatic RCC. Cytosol preparations were incubated with ³H-estradiol and analyzed by sucrose-density gradients. A single class of estrogen-binding sites was identified, which was inhibited by unlabeled estradiol, estriol, and estrone, but only weakly so by progesterone. There were 10 to 27 fmol of ³H-estradiol bound per milligram of cytosol protein; the dissociation constants were similar to those in human breast cancer and normal human kidney samples. It is not clear from this report whether ER was found in every sample, and the authors pointed out that the cell of origin of these ER proteins, whether stromal cells, normal tubule cells, or malignant "clear" or granular cells, is not known. Posey et al.[78] used similar sucrose-gradient techniques to demonstrate ER at levels greater than 6 fmol estradiol binding per milligram of cytosol protein in two of five RCC samples.

Agar gel electrophoresis and Scatchard plot analysis were used by Concolino et al.[62,63] to assay ER and PR receptor proteins in three normal-kidney and 10 RCC samples. One of the normal, and five of the RCC samples contained specific ER. The quantitative data suggested that RCC has a similar estrogen-binding capacity to normal kidney, but a higher capacity for progesterone.

C. Laboratory Models

Exogenous estrogens induce malignancy in a variety of animals, but the tumor sites differ with the species tested. In rats and mice, estrogen administration produces cancers of the breast, bladder, and pituitary;[40] guinea pigs develop peritoneal fibromas, lymphatic malignancies, and adrenal tumors, while rabbits develop endometrial carcinoma. In laboratory primates, no consistent estrogen-induced tumor has been shown. Only in hamsters does induction of renal malignancy occur with any frequency.[39]

Normal hamster kidney is an estrogen target tissue, with appreciable quantities of precipitable ER proteins,[75] measurable renal hypertrophy after exogenous estrogen,[15,80] and induction of esterase isoenzymes in castrated adult animals after stilbestrol treatment.[38] This contrasts with mouse and rat kidney, where estrogens induce renal atrophy.[15] Although hamsters may spontaneously develop malignant renal tumors, these tumors consist of undifferentiated spindle cells with a different enzyme pattern from that of the Kirkman stilbestrol-induced renal carcinoma.[81,82] In the latter model, subcutaneous implantation of pellets containing 20 mg of stilbestrol induces RCC in 70 to 80% of male, and 66% of castrated female hamsters, after a 9- to 12-month induction period (equal to one third of the hamster life span). Intact females do not develop these tumors, and different estrogen preparations vary in their ability to induce tumorigenesis.[83] The hamster's immunologic status does not significantly alter tumor growth or spread.[84]

Histologic studies show tumor multicentricity, with early alteration in the renal stroma, and the first nodules developing at the corticomedullary junction.[81,82] Tumors exhibit diverse histology, with areas showing blastemal, epithelial, or normal tubular appearance.[83] Electron microscopy reveals that cells become more ciliated, and intercellular gap junctions develop, as the dosage or duration of estrogen treatment increases.[85] Llombart-Bosch and Peydra[83] concluded from their histochemical studies that interstitial-cell hyperplasia was the origin of this neoplasm, and that no human renal carcinoma showed a close histologic similarity.

Horning[86] reported that 65% of hamsters developing primary Kirkman tumors also had pituitary pars intermedia tumors. Hamilton et al.[80] noted that stilbestrol caused a ten-fold increase in hamster pituitary weight, with hypertrophy and hyperplasia of prolactin-secreting cells. Although prolactin inhibitors allegedly protected animals from estrogen-induced renal tumors,[80] suggesting a role for prolactin in the neoplastic transformation, hypophysectomy had no effect on tumor development.

The Kirkman renal carcinoma does contain estrogen-receptor proteins, and is influenced by endogenous and exogenous estrogens. Li et al.[87] reported that estradiol-binding molecules in both hamster renal tumors and in uterus had similar sedimentation characteristics, affinity constants, and numbers of binding sites. After 12 to 20 serial passages to stilbestrol-primed recipients, the tumors acquire partial "stilbestrol autonomy", which first appears in focal clones of cells, such that they require only small amounts of endogenous estrogen for growth.[82] Both the primary and autonomous tumors retain similar isoenzyme banding patterns[81] and a similar number of estradiol binding sites with unchanged hormone affinity.[88] The "autonomous" tumors are inhibited by antiestrogens;[17,82] Kirkman[82] suggested that the transplants may synthesize their own estrogens, because they are associated with testicular atrophy in host male rats.

Cell cultures of the nonautonomous tumors have been maintained for up to five passages without any noticeable effect of stilbestrol on growth or morphology.[89] In vitro, the cells appeared fibroblastic, but in vivo they reinitiated hamster tumors in which most cells appeared to be epithelial in type. Even after 14 serial transplants, subcutaneous stilbestrol pellets were required for growth in vivo, while the estrogen was without effect on tumor explants in vitro. Similarly, Sirbasku and Kirkland[90] established a permanent epithelial cell line (H-301) from a Syrian hamster RCC, where in vivo tumor growth required exogenous estrogen; but, in vitro, growth was estrogen independent, and no specific uptake of ^{3}H-estradiol occurred.

Steggles and King[75,91] reviewed these data and concluded that there was no proven correlation between hormone dependency and estradiol-binding potency in the Kirkman tumor model, and that tumor induction might not involve a direct stilbestrol action on the hamster kidney target cell. Williams et al. [58] have expressed the view that the hamster renal carcinoma is not directly useful as a model for human RCC. Recently, other animal models for RCC have been described. Murphy and Hrushesky[64] reported a spontaneous renal carcinoma which developed in a male Balb/c Cr mouse. This tumor grew in syngeneic mice as a grey-white, vascular, invasive carcinoma with a granular-cell histology. It progressed equally well in both sexes, had a high mitotic rate with a 7-day doubling time, was transplantable by 10^5 tumor cells, and grew best when placed beneath the renal capsule. The tumor metastasized widely by day 14, and killed recipient animals by day 60. Tumor growth was accelerated by both exogenous testosterone and stilbestrol, but progestogens had no effect on growth rate.[64,92] Whether or not this tumor contains hormone-receptor proteins is unknown. However, the model does show some promise in screening of chemotherapeutic agents for efficacy in human RCC. Both vinblastine and CCNU appeared modestly active against this animal tumor, as they are against human renal carcinoma. Other agents, such as bleomycin, hydroxyurea, cyclophosphamide, and hexamethylmelamine have had equivocal activity in both species.[58,93,94]

Soloway and Myers[95] described another spontaneous renal carcinoma in a male Balb/cf/Cd mouse. This tumor (MKT-Cdl) was transplantable to both sexes with 10^4 cells, but stilbestrol pretreatment decreased the number of animals developing tumors. Both testosterone and stilbestrol had a slightly inhibitory effect on tumor growth, but, like the previous model, MPA at a dose of 10 to 25 mg/kg had little effect on tumor induction or growth.

There are few in vitro data regarding the effect of estrogens on human RCC tissue. Tchao et al.[44] reported growth suppression by stilbestrol in five of six tumor explants, but Card et al.[45] noted no estrogenic effect on six samples similarly tested. Further in vitro studies, correlating histological chanes induced by estrogens and antiestrogens with tissue ER and PR status, would be of interest.

D. Clinical Results

The facts that human RCC occurs twice as often in men as in women, and that men receiving stilbestrol for prostatic cancer have no increased incidence of RCC, argue against estrogen induction of this tumor.[3] Kinlen et al.[96] reported a British study in which questionnaires were sent to physicians regarding stilbestrol prescriptions to pregnant women during the prior 30 years. Although an estimated 7500 women received stilbestrol, and approximately 4500 received other estrogens during this period (1940 to 1971), the incidence of carcinoma of the kidney, ureter, and renal pelvis remained unchanged.

Legha and Muggia[97] reported two complete and one partial remission, induced by treatment with the antiestrogen nafoxidine, in 20 patients with RCC. They also referred to unpublished data in which two of four patients responded to the antiestrogen tamoxifen. However, a recently completed, as yet unpublished, study by the Southwest Oncology Group tested tamoxifen effect in 35 patients with metastatic renal-cell carcinoma.[101] The agent was given orally as 10 mg twice daily, for at least 6 weeks. Toxicity was minimal, but only two partial responses were reported in 35 evaluable cases. However, eleven other patients had no change noted in their disease during treatment, and tamoxifen may still have some useful therapeutic role in RCC.

E. Summary

Although exogenous estrogens induce a variety of tumors in animals, there is no common pattern of tumor induction, and the hamster is the only animal where renal cancer consistently occurs. There are no current data showing that the hamster model is applicable to human renal carcinoma, and stilbestrol induction and growth promotion in this model may occur through an indirect metabolic effect. There are no data to suggest that estrogen induces renal carcinoma in man.

Although specific estrogen-receptor proteins have been identified in both normal kidney and renal carcinoma tissues, these receptor data have not yet been correlated with the therapeutic response of patients treated with antiestrogens or with other endocrine manipulations. Further study of estrogen receptors in renal carcinoma tissue, coupled with clinical trials of antiestrogens, castration, or medical adrenalectomy, may be useful approaches to palliating this malignancy.

V. GLUCOCORTICOIDS IN RENAL-CELL CARCINOMA

Although glucocorticoid receptors are found in a variety of nonlymphoid tissues,[27] there are no reports describing these proteins in normal or malignant renal tissue. Because of a general inhibitory effect on DNA, RNA and protein synthesis, and decreased capillary proliferation,[51] one might expect some glucocorticoid activity against metastatic renal carcinoma. However, Card et al.[45] found no consistent effect of hydrocortisone on 10 human RCC explants in vitro. Both Talley et al.[14] and Lokich and Harrison[54] reported a complete lack of therapeutic response to corticosteroids in a total of 51 patients. Similar negative results were obtained at the University of Wisconsin. When nine patients were treated with prednisone, at an average dose of 45 mg per day for an average of 1.2 months, none, including several who also received cytotoxic drugs, showed an objective response. Neither did three others given other corticosteroids.[22]

Thus, although glucocorticoids may produce a few objective responses in breast cancer, and might have a palliative role in RCC, there is no evidence that they have a significant direct antitumor effect.

VI. CONCLUSION

Although the Kirkman renal carcinoma in the Syrian hamster has been invoked to justify hormonal therapy of human RCC, it is clear that this model is more complex than originally thought, and is not directly applicable to the human situation. Further blind hormonal maneuvers involving individual patients in a nonstudy environment are unlikely to be productive, and cannot be justified, given the current plethora of negative hormonal data.

Perhaps the clinical dictum, "hypernephroma is resistant to chemotherapy" has encouraged physicians to attempt hormonal therapy for want of a viable alternative. Yet Carter and Wasserman[98] identified only two chemotherapeutic agents which had been adequately evaluated, and Hrushesky and Murphy[99] noted that only vinblastine has been used in more than 100 patients. Thus, properly designed chemotherapy trials must take a higher priority in future studies of RCC treatment. Further hormonal approaches to human RCC might benefit from:

1. Careful definition of hormone receptor status in the resected tumor.
2. In vitro metabolic studies, including autoradiography, to define the cell population retaining the hormone.
3. Patient endocrine profiling while hormone/antihormone is being administered; to help separate direct from indirect hormonal effects.

4. Careful tumor staging and use of standardized response criteria, while bearing in mind that hormone-responsive tumors may respond to hormonal manipulation differently at different metastatic sites.[100]
5. Careful attention to patient survival, with either comparison to a matched historical control or, optimally, to a prospectively randomized, hormone-untreated cohort.
6. Continued search for useful animal and cell-culture models.

We conclude and concur with Bloom's 1963 assessment of the problem, " . . . more work needs to be done before one can speak of hormone-dependency in human renal carcinoma."[15]

ACKNOWLEDGMENTS

The author thanks Felipe B. Manalo, M.D. and Ms. Debbie Powers for assistance in reviewing the University of Wisconsin clinical material. He would also like to thank Ms. Jane Harberg for help with data management.

REFERENCES

1. **Frank, I. N.**, Urologic and male genital cancers, in *Clinical Oncology*, 4th ed., Rubin, P. and Bakemeier, R. F., Eds., American Cancer Society, New York, 1974, 258.
2. **Silverberg, E.**, *Urologic Cancer Statistical and Epidemiological Information*, American Cancer Society, New York, 1973, 10.
3. **Bloom, H. J. G.**, Renal Cancer, in *Endocrine Therapy in Malignant Disease*, Stoll, B. A., Ed., W. B. Saunders, London, 1972, 339.
4. **Marlow, P. B. and Mizel, S.**, Evidence for rhythm of mitotic activity in normal and adenocarcinoma cells of the renal tubules of *Rana pipiens*, *J. Natl. Cancer Inst.*, 57, 1069, 1976.
5. **Holland, J. M.**, Cancer of the kidney — natural history and staging, *Cancer (Philadelphia)*, 32, 1030, 1973.
6. **Murphy, G. P., Kenny, G. M., and Mirand, E. A.**, Erythropoietin levels in patients with renal tumors or cysts, *Cancer (Philadelphia)*, 26, 191, 1970.
7. **Ellis, D. J.**, Hormones and the kidney, *Br. J. Urol.*, 48, 153, 1976.
8. **Sufrin, G., Mirand, E. A., Moore, R. H., Chu, T. M., and Murphy, G. P.**, Hormones in renal cancer, *J. Urol.*, 117, 433, 1977.
9. **Sherwood, J. B. and Goldwasser, E.**, Erythropoietin production by human renal carcinoma cells in culture, *Endocrinology*, 99, 504, 1976.
10. **Gibbons, R. P., Montie, J. E., Correa, R. J., and Mason, J. T.**, Manifestations of renal cell carcinoma, *Urology*, 8, 201, 1976.
11. **Schellhammer, P. F. and Smith, M. J. V.**, Renal cell carcinoma in children, *South. Med. J.*, 66, 1345, 1973.
12. **Bloom, H. J. G.**, Cancer of the urogenital tract: kidney. The basis for hormonal therapy, *JAMA*, 204, 605, 1968.
13. **Bloom, H. J. G.**, Adjuvant therapy for adenocarcinoma of the kidney: present position and prospects, *Br. J. Urol.*, 45, 237, 1973.
14. **Talley, R. W., Moorhead, E. L., Tucker, W. G., San Diego, E. L., and Brennan, M. J.**, Treatment of metastatic hypernephroma, *JAMA*, 207, 322, 1969.
15. **Bloom, H. J. G., Dukes, C. E., and Mitchley, B. G. V.**, The oestrogen-induced renal tumor of the Syrian hamster. Hormone treatment and possible relationship to carcinoma of the kidney in man, *Br. J. Cancer*, 17, 611, 1963.
16. **Bloom, H. J. G., Baker, W. H., Dukes, C. E., and Mitchley, B. C. V.**, Effect of endocrine ablation procedures on the transplanted oestrogen-induced renal tumor of the Syrian hamster, *Br. J. Cancer*, 17, 646, 1963.

17. **Bloom, H. J. G., Roe, F. J., and Mitchley, B. C. V.**, Sex hormones and renal neoplasia. Inhibition of tumor of hamster kidney by an estrogen antagonist, an agent of possible therapeutic value in man, *Cancer (Philadelphia)*, 20, 2118, 1967.
18. **Bloom, H. J. G.**, Medroxyprogesterone acetate (Provera) in the treatment of metastatic renal cancer, *Br. J. Cancer*, 25, 250, 1971.
19. **Bloom, H. J. G.**, Adjuvant therapy for adenocarcinoma of the kidney: present position and prospects, *Br. J. Urol.*, 45, 237, 1973.
20. **Bloom, H. J. G.**, Proceedings: hormone-induced and spontaneous regression of metastatic renal cancer, *Cancer (Philadelphia)*, 32, 1066, 1973.
21. **Van der Werf-Messing, B. and Van Gilse, H. A.**, Hormonal treatment of metastases of renal carcinoma, *Br. J. Cancer*, 25, 423, 1971.
22. **Hogan, T. F.**, Unpublished data, 1978.
23. **Böttiger, L. E. and Lisboa, B. P.**, 17-Ketosteroid excretion in renal carcinoma, *Clin. Chim. Acta*, 16, 109, 1967.
24. **Bojar, H., Funcke, C., Dreyfurst, R., Matthiesen, U., and Staib, W.**, Testosterone metabolism of isolated human kidney tubules, *Horm. Metab. Res.*, 9, 252, 1977.
25. **Sluyser, M.**, Interaction of steroid hormones and histones, in *The Biochemistry of Steroid Hormone Action*, Smellie, R. M. S., Ed., Academic Press, New York, 1971, 31.
26. **Liao, S.**, Biochemical studies on the receptor mechanism involved in androgen actions, in *Biochemistry of Hormones*, Vol. 8, Rickenberg, H. V., Ed., University Park Press, Baltimore, 1972, 153.
27. **Liao, S., Hung, S. C., Tymocyko, J. L., and Liang, T.**, Active forms and biodynamics of the androgen-receptor in various target tissues, in *Steroid Hormone Action and Cancer*, Menon, K. M. J. and Reel, J. R., Eds., Plenum Press, New York, 1974, 139.
28. **Rennie, P. and Bruchovsky, N.**, Effect of binding proteins on androgen localization in target tissues, in *Proc. 4th Int. Cong. Endocrinology*, Excerpta Medica Foundation, Amsterdam, 1972, 79.
29. **Marberger, M., Jr., Altwein, J. E., and Orestano, F.**, The influence of the progestogen gestonorone caproate on testosterone turnover in renal cell carcinoma. An in vitro study, *Invest. Urol.*, 13, 302, 1976.
30. **Goldenberg, I. S. and Segaloff, A.**, Principles of endocrine therapy: androgens, in *Cancer Medicine*, Holland, J. F. and Frei, E., Eds., Lea & Febiger, Philadelphia, 1973, 931.
31. **Ritzen, E. M., Nayfeh, S. N., French, F. S., and Aronin, P. A.**, Deficient nuclear uptake of testosterone in the androgen-insensitive (Stanley-Gumbreck) pseudohermaphrodite male rat, *Endocrinology*, 91, 116, 1972.
32. **Gehring, U., Tomkins, G. M., and Ohno, S.**, Effect of the androgen-insensitivity mutation on a cytoplasmic receptor for dihydrotestosterone, *Nature (London), New Biol.*, 232, 106, 1971.
33. **McCarty, K. S., Jr. and McCarty, K. S., Sr.**, Steroid hormone receptors in the regulation of differentiation, *Am. J. Pathol.*, 86, 705, 1977.
34. **Bullock, L. P. and Bordin, C. W.**, Androgen receptors in mouse kidney: a study of male, female, and androgen-insensitive (tfm/y) mice, *Endocrinology*, 94, 746, 1974.
35. **Fanestil, D. D., Vaughn, D. A., and Ludens, J. H.**, Steroid hormone receptors in human renal carcinoma, *J. Steroid Biochem.*, 5, 338, 1974.
36. **Murad, F. and Gilman, A. G.**, Androgens and anabolic steroids, in *The Pharmacologic Basis of Therapeutics*, 5th ed., Goodman, L. S. and Gilman, A., Eds., Macmillan, New York, 1975, 1459.
37. **Noronha, R. F. X.**, The inhibition of dimethylnitrosamine induced renal tumorigenesis in NZO/Bl mice by orchidectomy, *Invest. Urol.*, 13, 136, 1975.
38. **Li, J. J., Kirkman, H., and Hunter, R. L.**, Sex difference and gonadal hormone influence on Syrian hamster kidney esterase isozymes, *J. Histochem. Cytochem.*, 17, 386, 1969.
39. **Segaloff, A.**, Steroids and carcinogenesis, *J. Steroid. Biochem.*, 6, 171, 1975.
40. **Noble, R. L., Hochachka, B. C., and King, D.**, Spontaneous and estrogen-produced tumors in NB rats and their behavior after transplantation, *Cancer Res.*, 35, 766, 1975.
41. **Weisburger, J. H., Griswold, D. P., Prejean, J. D., Casey, A. E., Wood, H. B., and Weisburger, E. K.**, The carcinogenic properties of some of the principal drugs used in clinical cancer chemotherapy, in *Recent Reports in Cancer Research: The Ambivalence of Cytostatic Therapy*, Grundmann, E. and Gross, R., Eds., Springer-Verlag, New York, 1975, 1.
42. **Roe, F. J., Boyland, E., Dukes, C. E., and Mitchley, B. C.**, Failure of testosterone or xanthopterin to influence the induction of renal neoplasms by lead in rats, *Br. J. Cancer*, 19, 860, 1965.
43. **Kaufman, J. J.**, Cancer of the kidney: diagnostic, therapeutic, and experimental vistas, the Percy T. Magan Memorial Lecture, 1973, *Med. Arts Sci.*, 27, 28, 1973.
44. **Tchao, R., Easty, G. C., Ambrose, E. J., Raven, R. W., and Bloom, H. J. G.**, Effect of chemotherapeutic agents and hormones on organ cultures of human tumors, *Eur. J. Cancer*, 4, 39, 1968.
45. **Card, D. J., Kohorn, E. I., and Lyttun, B.**, Effects of hormones on whole organ cultures of renal cell carcinoma, *Surg. Forum*, 21, 532, 1970.

46. **Jenkin, R. D.,** Androgens in metastatic renal adenocarcinoma, *Br. Med. J.,* 1, 361, 1967.
47. **Samuels, M. L., Sullivan, P., and Howe, C. D.,** Medroxyprogesterone acetate in the treatment of renal cell carcinoma (hypernephroma), *Cancer (Philadelphia),* 22, 525, 1968.
48. **Papec, R. J.,** Hormonal therapy of renal carcinoma, in *Proceedings of the American Association of Cancer Research, Vol. 10,* Shimkin, M. B. and Kravitz, E., Eds., Goodway, Philadelphia, 1969, 67.
49. **Paine, C. H., Wright, F. W., and Ellis, F.,** The use of progestogen in the treatment of metastatic carcinoma of the kidney and uterine body, *Br. J. Cancer,* 24, 277, 1970.
50. **Wagle, D. G. and Murphy, G. P.,** Hormonal therapy in advanced renal cell carcinoma, *Cancer (Philadelphia),* 28, 318, 1971.
51. **Talley, R. W.,** Proceedings: Chemotherapy of adenocarcinoma of the kidney, *Cancer (Philadelphia),* 32, 1062, 1973.
52. **Alberto, P. and Senn, H. J.,** Hormonal therapy of renal carcinoma alone and in association with cytostatic drugs, *Cancer (Philadelphia),* 33, 1226, 1974.
53. **Morales, A., Kiruluta, G., and Lott, S.,** Hormones in the treatment of metastatic renal cancer, *J. Urol.,* 114, 692, 1975.
54. **Lokich, J. J. and Harrison, J. H.,** Renal cell carcinoma: natural history and chemotherapeutic experience, *J. Urol.,* 114, 371, 1975.
55. **Papec, R. J., Ross, S. A., and Levy, A.,** Renal cell carcinoma: analysis of 31 cases with assessment of endocrine therapy, *Am. J. Med. Sci.,* 274, 281, 1977.
56. **Kelley, R. M.,** Principles of endocrine therapy: progestins, in *Cancer Medicine,* Holland, J. F. and Frei, E., Eds., Lea & Febiger, Philadelphia, 1973, 925.
57. **Hellman, L., Yoshida, K., Zumoff, B., Levin, J., Kream, J., and Fukushima, D. K.,** The effect of medroxyprogesterone acetate on the pituitary-adrenal axis, *J. Clin. Endocrinol. Metab.,* 42, 912, 1976.
58. **Williams, P. D., Burdick, J., and Murphy, G. P.,** Evaluation of hexamethylmelamine in murine renal cell carcinoma model, *Res. Commun. Chem. Pathol. Pharmacol.,* 7, 400, 1974.
59. **Sadoff, L. and Lusk, W.,** The effect of large doses of medroxyprogesterone acetate (MPA) on urinary estrogen levels and serum levels of cortisol, T_4, LH, and testosterone in patients with advanced cancer, *Obstet. Gynecol.,* 43, 262, 1974.
60. **Faber, L. E., Saffran, J., Chen, T. J., and Leavitt, W. W.,** Mammalian progesterone receptors: biosynthesis, structure, and nuclear binding, in *Steroid Hormone Action and Cancer,* Menon, K. M. J. and Reel, J. R., Eds., Plenum Press, New York, 1974, 68.
61. **Pasqualini, J. R., Sumida, C., and Gelly, C.,** Steroid hormone receptors in fetal guinea pig kidney, *J. Steroid Biochem.,* 5, 977, 1974.
62. **Concolino, G., Marocchi, A., Concolino, F., Sciarra, F., Di Silverio, F., and Conti, C.,** Human kidney steroid receptors, *J. Steroid Biochem.,* 7, 831, 1976.
63. **Concolino, G., Marocchi, A., Di Silverio, F., and Conti, C.,** Progestational therapy in human renal carcinoma and steroid receptors, *J. Steroid Biochem.,* 7, 923, 1976.
64. **Murphy, G. P. and Hrushesky, W. J.,** A murine renal cell carcinoma, *J. Natl. Cancer Inst.,* 50, 1013, 1973.
65. **Woodruff, M. W., Wagle, D., Gailani, S. D., and Jones, R., Jr.,** The current status of chemotherapy for advanced renal carcinoma, *J. Urol.,* 97, 611, 1967.
66. **Melander, O., Notter, G., and von Schreeb, T.,** Hormonbehandling av metastaserande renal kancer, *Nordisk Med.,* 5, 1309, 1967.
67. **Ramirez, G., Weiss, A. J., Rochlin, D. B., and Bisel, H. F.,** Phase II study of 6α-methylpreg-4-ene-3,11,20 trione, *Cancer Chemother. Rep.,* 55, 265, 1971.
68. **Murnaghan, G.,** Endocrine aspects of renal carcinoma, *Br. J. Urol.,* 44, 126, 1972.
69. **Johnson, D. E. and Samuels, M. L.,** Chemotherapy of metastatic renal carcinoma, in *Cancer Chemotherapy: Fundamental Concepts and Recent Advances, Annual Clinical Conference on Cancer,* M. D. Anderson Hospital and Tumor Institute, Year Book Medical Publishing, Chicago, 1975, 493.
70. **Peterson, L. J., Grimes, J. H., Dees, J. E., and Anderson, E. E.,** Hormonal therapy in metastatic hypernephroma, *Urology,* 4, 669, 1974.
71. **Hahn, R. G.,** Controlled Phase II Studies in the Treatment of Advanced Renal Cancer, Eastern Cooperative Oncology Group Report, EST 1874, Madison, Wisconsin, 1976.
72. **Hahn, R. G., Temkin, N. R., Savlov, E. O., Perlia, C., Wampler, G. L., Horton, J., Marsh, J., and Carbone, P. P.,** Phase II study of vinblastine, methyl-CCNU, medroxyprogesterone in advanced renal cell carcinoma, *Cancer Treatment Rep.,* 62, 1093, 1978.
73. **Wynder, E. L., Mabuchi, K., and Whitmore, W. F., Jr.,** Epidemiology of adenocarcinoma of the kidney, *J. Natl. Cancer Inst.,* 53, 1619, 1974.
74. **Lemon, H. M.,** Principles of endocrine therapy: estrogens in *Cancer Medicine,* Holland, J. F. and Frei, E., Eds., Lea & Febiger, Philadelphia, 1973, 911.

75. **Steggles, A. W. and King, R. J.**, Oestrogen receptors in hamster tumours, *Eur. J. Cancer,* 8, 323, 1972.
76. **DeVries, J. R., Ludens, J. H., and Fanestil, D. D.**, Estradiol renal receptors and estradiol-dependent antinatriuresis, *Kidney Int.,* 2, 95, 1972.
77. **Bojar, H., Dreyfurst, R., Balzer, K., Staib, W., and Wittliff, J. L.**, Oestrogen-binding components in human renal cell carcinoma, *J. Clin. Chem. Clin. Biochem.,* 14, 521, 1976.
78. **Posey, L. E., Morgan, L. R., Beayley, R. M., Lanasa, J., Torres, J., Krementy, E. T., Carter, R. D., Sutherland, C., and Hawley, W.**, Estrogen receptors, *JAMA,* 238, 2599, 1977.
79. **Freifeld, M. L., Feil, P. D., and Bardin, C. W.**, The in vitro regulation of the progesterone "receptor" in guinea pig uterus: dependence on estrogen and progesterone, *Steroids,* 23, 93, 1974.
80. **Hamilton, J. M., Saluja, P. G., Thody, A. J., and Flaks, A.**, The pars intermedia and renal carcinogenesis in hamsters, *Eur. J. Cancer,* 13, 29, 1977.
81. **Kirkman, H.**, Hormone-related tumors in Syrian hamsters, *Prog. Exp. Tumor Res.,* 16, 201, 1972.
82. **Kirkman, H.**, Autonomous derivatives of estrogen-induced renal carcinomas and spontaneous renal tumors in the Syrian hamster, *Cancer Res.,* 34, 2728, 1974.
83. **Llombart-Bosch, A. and Peydra, A.**, Morphologic, histochemical, and ultrastructural observations of diethylstilbestrol-induced kidney tumors in the Syrian golden hamster, *Eur. J. Cancer,* 2, 403, 1975.
84. **McLaughlin, A. P., III, Kessler, W. O., and Gittes, B. F.**, The dissociation between endocrine carcinogenesis and tumor antigenicity, *Invest. Urol.,* 12, 83, 1974.
85. **LeFourneau, P. J., Li, J. J., Rosen, S., and Villee, C. A.**, Junctional specialization in estrogen-induced renal adenocarcinomas of the golden hamster, *Cancer Res.,* 35, 6, 1975.
86. **Horning, E. S.**, Hormonal neoplasia: tumors induced with oestrogen and androgen, *Br. Emp. Cancer Campaign Ann. Rep.,* 33, 62, 1955.
87. **Li, J. J., Talley, D. J., Li, S. A., and Villee, C. A.**, Receptor characteristics of specific estrogen binding in the renal adenocarcinoma of the golden hamster, *Cancer Res.,* 36, 1127, 1976.
88. **King, R. J., Smith, J. A., and Steggles, A. W.**, Oestrogen-binding and the hormone responsiveness of tumours, *Steroidologia,* 1, 73, 1970.
89. **Dekernion, J. B. and Fraley, E. E.**, Growth characteristics of the stilbestrol-induced hamster kidney tumor, *J. Surg. Oncol.,* 3, 507, 1971.
90. **Sirbasku, D. A., and Kirkland, W. L.**, Control of cell growth. IV. Growth properties of a new cell line established from an estrogen-dependent kidney tumor of the Syrian hamster, *Endocrinology,* 98, 1260, 1976.
91. **Steggles, A. W. and King, R. J.**, The uptake of (16, 7—³H) oestradiol by oestrogen dependent and independent hamster kidney tumours, *Eur. J. Cancer,* 4, 395, 1968.
92. **Williams, P. D., Bhanalaph, T., and Murphy, G. P.**, Unilateral nephrectomy, its effect on primary murine renal cell adenocarcinoma, *Urology,* 2, 619, 1973.
93. **Hrushesky, W. J. and Murphy, G. P.**, Evaluation of chemotherapy agents in a new murine renal carcinoma model, *J. Natl. Cancer Inst.,* 52, 1117, 1974.
94. **Schefner, A. M. and Marlow, M.**, Preliminary drug trials in a renal cell carcinoma animal model, *Cancer Chemother. Rep.,* 5, 145, 1975.
95. **Soloway, M. S. and Myers, G. H., Jr.**, The effect of hormonal therapy on a transplantable renal cortical adenocarcinoma in syngeneic mice, *J. Urol.,* 109, 356, 1973.
96. **Kinlen, L. J., Badaracco, M. A., Moffett, J., and Vessey, M. P.**, A survey of the use of oestrogens during pregnancy in the United Kingdom and of the genito-urinary cancer mortality and incidence rates in young people in England and Wales, *J. Obstet. Gynaecol. Br. Emp.,* 81, 849, 1974.
97. **Legha, S. and Muggia, F. M.**, Antiestrogens in the treatment of cancer, *Ann. Int. Med.,* 84, 751, 1976.
98. **Carter, S. K. and Wasserman, T. H.**, The chemotherapy of urologic cancer, *Cancer (Philadelphia),* 36, 729, 1975.
99. **Hrushesky, W. J. and Murphy, G. P.**, Current status of the therapy of advanced renal carcinoma, *J. Surg. Oncol.,* 9, 277, 1977.
100. **Noble, R. L.**, Hormonal control of growth and progression in tumors of NB rats and a theory of action, *Cancer Res.,* 37, 82, 1977.
101. **Al Sarraf, M.**, Phase II Study of Tamifoxen in Metastatic Renal Cell Carcinoma, Southwest Oncology Group Report, SWOG, 77-16, Kansas City, Kansas, September, 1978.

Chapter 4

ENDOCRINE ASPECTS OF MALIGNANT MELANOMA

Richard I. Fisher and Marc E. Lippman

TABLE OF CONTENTS

I. INTRODUCTION

Scientific investigation into the biologic behavior of malignant melanoma may appear excessive in view of the fact that malignant melanoma is an uncommon tumor, constituting only 1 to 3% of all human cancer.[1] Yet certain aspects of the natural history of this disease have suggested that malignant melanoma might provide an interesting model for the study of host and tumor interactions. The reports of antitumor immunity in some patients with melanoma[2] and the finding that melanoma is one of the most common tumors to undergo spontaneous regression[3] have suggested that melanoma could be studied as a model for the immunologic control of human neoplasia. Malignant melanoma is not usually considered to be a hormone-dependent tumor. Until recently very limited consideration has been given to those aspects of the natural history of malignant melanoma that suggest that hormonal influences might be important in the induction or growth of this neoplasm. There are, however, some epidemiologic data to support this contention. We have previously demonstrated that steroid hormone receptor activity can be detected in a significant number of human melanomas. A clinical trial has been instituted to determine whether these receptors can be correlated with certain aspects of the natural history of melanoma and whether endocrine manipulation could be utilized as an effective therapy for a subset of patients with malignant melanoma.

II. HISTORICAL DATA SUGGESTING HORMONAL INFLUENCE

A. Epidemiology

Human malignant melanoma is an extremely rare disease before puberty. From a population base of approximately 3 million in southwest England, Bodenham and Hale recorded only one case of malignant melanoma in a patient under the age of 13 and one case in the age range of 13 to 15 during a 10-year period.[4] The overall incidence of melanoma in that population was 3.5 cases per 100,000 population per year. McGovern's series of 202 patients describing the natural history of melanoma in New South Wales, Australia, included only 2 patients below the age of 15.[5] Furthermore, Pack and Scharnagel reported that in a series of 1050 verified cases, they had never seen a case of melanoma in infancy or childhood with metastases or a fatal outcome.[6] For female patients the highest risk of developing malignant melanoma coincides with the childbearing years.[4] However a second peak of high incidence can also be observed in the postmenopausal ages, from 60 to 70 years. Although there has been considerable variation in reports concerning the relative incidence of malignant melanoma in males vs. females, there is no controversy regarding the fact that the prognosis in females is significantly better than males. The increased survival of females relative to males has been documented regardless of stage or treatment.[7,8]

B. Pregnancy and Melanoma

The effects of pregnancy on the natural history of malignant melanoma are more controversial than any other aspect of data that suggest some endocrine regulation of melanoma. Initial concern about the effect of pregnancy was caused by early case reports of rapid dissemination of melanoma during pregnancy.[9] In 1957, Pack and Scharnagel from Memorial Hospital, New York reported that 32 patients in whom the diagnosis of malignant melanoma had been made just prior to, during, or immediately following a pregnancy had a short survival;[6] thus these authors conclude that pregnancy had an adverse effect on the course of melanoma. The concept that pregnancy had an adverse effect on the prognosis of melanoma was further supported by reports of spontaneous regression of melanoma following partuition. Allen reported a case of melanoma in which multiple skin metastases developed during pregnancy;[10] all tumor regressed within 2 months of delivery and the patient was disease-free 12 years later. Byrd reported a patient whose melanoma grew during each of five pregnancies and then regressed during each postpartum period.[11]

When larger series of pregnant patients were studied and compared to nonpregnant patients with melanoma, most authors concluded that pregnancy did not have an adverse effect on the course of malignant melanoma. The experience at Memorial Sloan Kettering Hospital was reviewed again in 1960 by George et al.[12] A group of 115 patients who were pregnant sometime during the course of melanoma were compared to a group of 330 nonpregnant female controls. The 5- and 10-year survival rates for the two groups were essentially the same. A small group of pregnant patients with Stage II disease did appear to have a shorter survival than matched controls but the numbers were too small for statistical analysis. These authors' conclusions that pregnancy did not exert an adverse effect on the course of melanoma were also supported by White et al.[13] They found no difference in survival between 31 nonpregnant melanoma patients and 30 patients whose pregnancy occurred from 1 year before diagnosis to 5 years following diagnosis. However, neither of these last two papers provided documentation that all known prognostic factors were equally distributed in the pregnant and control patients. The experience at Memorial Hospital was reviewed a third time in 1976 by Shiu et al.[14] A group of 251 Stage I or II female patients were classified as nulliparous, parous but without changes in a suspected lesion during the previous pregnancy, parous with definite changes in a suspected lesion during previous pregnancy, and pregnant during therapy. There was no difference in survival for Stage I patients in any of these groups. However, the 5-year survival of Stage II patients who were pregnant during therapy or had activation of a suspected lesion during a previous pregnancy was significantly less than that of the other two groups. This remains the only published study that has sufficient numbers of patients to determine the effect of melanoma on comparably staged pregnant patients.

C. Hormonal Therapy

Speculation that the growth of malignant melanoma might be influenced by hormones has been increased by occasional reports of patients with melanoma responding to hormonal therapies. Bodenham reported four patients treated with hormonal therapy (one with estrogens, one with androgens, and two with hypophysectomy) who showed dramatic tumor regressions of subcutaneous or lymph node metastases following treatment.[4] Johnson et al. reported at 11% objective response rate in patients with metastatic disease treated with 6 α-methylpregn-4-ene-3,11,20-trione, a drug with glucocorticoid and antiestrogen activity. However many other attempts at hormonal therapy have been unsuccessful. Howes described a male patient with extensive visceral disease who failed to respond to orchiectomy.[16] In a review article concerning the treatment of melanoma, Meyer and Gumport concluded that estrogens, androgens, pituitary irradiation, castration, and bilaterial adrenalectomy had been of no value.[17] However no details concerning the number of patients treated, extent of disease, etc. were reported. The latter conclusion was also supported by work at Memorial Hospital in 1951 when Pack and Scharnagel reported that castration, or testosterone therapy, had no beneficial effect on patients. Once again, the details of this study were not provided.[6] Although it is difficult to draw firm conclusions from such anecdotal case reports, the above data suggest that there may be a subset of patients with malignant melanoma who are responsive to hormone manipulation, although the majority of patients will not respond to such therapy.

III. STEROID HORMONE RECEPTORS

Because of the preceding data which suggested that hormones might affect the behavior of human malignant melanoma, studies were initiated by the Medicine and Surgery Branches of the National Cancer Institute to analyze tumor biopsies for the presence of cytoplasmic hormone receptors. In 1976 Fisher et al. reported that 16 of 35 tumor samples from patients (46%) with malignant melanoma had detectable estrogen receptor activity.[18] The cytosol from the tumor biopsies was assayed for estrogen receptor activity using modifications[19] of a previously described competitive protein-binding assay[20] in which dextran-coated charcoal was used to separate unbound [³H] estradiol-17β from protein-associated activity. This assay has been shown not to be confounded by estradiol binding to transport proteins. Since the biologic significance of these receptors in malignant melanoma is totally unknown, a positive assay was defined as one in which estrogen binding greater than the limits of detection of the assay, i.e., $\sim$ 5 fmol/mg cytoplasmic protein was found. Whenever sufficient amounts of tissue were available, Scatchard plots of binding data were also prepared.[21] A typical binding curve is shown in Figure 1 in which specific (competitive) binding is plotted as a function of increasing [³H] estradiol-17β concentration. The same binding data are replotted in the inset of this figure using the Scatchard technique. The straight line obtained (r = −0.82) suggests that under our assay conditions estradiol is binding to

BINDING OF (^{3}H)-ESTRADIOL TO HUMAN MELANOMA

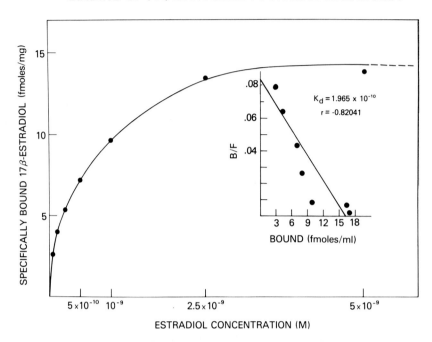

FIGURE 1.   Binding of [^{3}H]-estradiol to human melanoma. Cytosol extracts of melanoma were incubated in the presence of varying concentrations of 17β - estradiol and 1000-
fold excess of unlabeled estradiol. The data are replotted in the inset using the Scatchard
technique; the free steroid concentration is calculated by subtracting the bound steroid
from the amount added initially.

a class of receptor sites of uniform affinity and limited capacity. From the slope of
this line we estimate the dissociation constant to be 2×10^{-10} *M*. The "X" intercept
provides an estimation of the total number of receptor sites at saturating concentration
of steroid, in this case 24.7 fmol [^{3}H] estradiol bound per milligram of cytoplasmic
protein. When analyzed according to sex of the patients, 9 of 19 males (47%) and 7
of 16 females (43%) had estrogen receptor activity. Estrogen receptors were detected
in 2 of 3 biopsies of primary melanoma, 9 of 18 biopsies of lymph node metastases, 4
of 12 biopsies of skin metastases, and 1 of 2 biopsies of visceral metastases suggesting
that the presence of the estrogen receptor was not correlated with the specific site of
tumor biopsy.

The series of estrogen receptor assays in patients with malignant melanoma has now
been expanded to 77 patients. To date, 26 of 77 patients (34%) have detectable estrogen
receptors. The distribution of estrogen binding in malignant melanoma according to
the total number of receptor sites detected is shown in Figure 2. For most patients
with detectable estrogen receptors, the number of binding sites ranged from 5 to 35
fmol/mg cytoplasmic proteins. Very few patients had binding greater than 35 fmol/
mg cytoplasmic protein. These values are far lower than those found in samples analyzed from a group of patients with metastatic breast cancer.

We have also performed steroid receptor assays to detect progesterone and androgen
binding in melanoma tissues. Progesterone binding was assayed using a similar dextran-coated charcoal assay while 5α-dihydrotestosterone binding was determined with
a protamine sulfate assay.[19] The limits of sensitivity of the assays are 10 fmol/mg

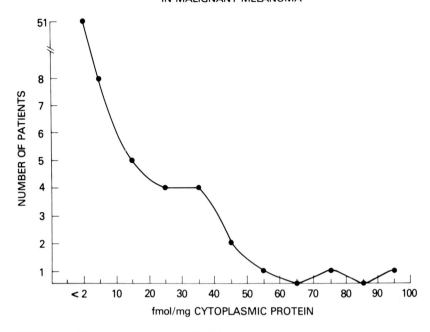

DISTRIBUTION OF ESTROGEN BINDING
IN MALIGNANT MELANOMA

FIGURE 2.   Distribution of estrogen binding in malignant melanoma. The number of patients with a given quantity of cytoplasmic estrogen binding sites is shown.

cytoplasmic protein for progesterone and 3 to 5 mg/cytoplasmic protein for androgens. For the reasons outlined above, steroid binding greater than the limits of detection of the assay has been defined as a positive result. Scatchard plots were again performed whenever sufficient tumor was available. We have detected progesterone binding in 19 of 58 patients (33%) and androgen binding in 15 of 57 patients (26%). There was no tendency demonstrated for the progesterone or androgen receptors to be linked to the estrogen receptor.

None of the binding components have been subjected to rigorous characterization by other techniques (e.g., sucrose density or agar gel electrophoresis) or detailed specificity studies. For these reasons it is probably not completely justified to refer to these binding components as "receptors". However, the use of 5α-dihydrotestosterone in competed and uncompeted tubes in the estrogen receptor assays, protamine sulfate precipitation for androgen receptor assays, and R5020 for progesterone receptor assays allows confidence that binding is not to plasma transport proteins.

IV. CLINICAL TRIALS OF HORMONE THERAPY

In 1976 we initiated a Phase II study of estrogen therapy for disseminated malignant melanoma.[22] In addition to determining the objective response rate to estrogen therapy, the study was designed to correlate objective responses with hormone receptor analyses in an attempt to define a subset of estrogen responsive patients. Eligibility criteria were as follows: (1) surgically nonresectable melanoma which could be biopsied for hormone receptors (however the results of the receptor analysis were never utilized as a selection criteria for the study), (2) clinically measurable disease, and (3) males or postmenopausal females. Premenopausal females were not included in the study be-

TABLE 1

DES Therapy for Malignant Melanoma: Patient Characteristics

Total patients	24
Sex	
Males	21
Females	3
Median age (Range)	37 (17—62)
Sites of disease	
Soft tissue plus	5
lymph nodes only	
Visceral metastases	19
Prior therapy	
Chemotherapy	18
Immunotherapy	9
Median Karnofsky rating (range)	80 (50—100)

cause of some concern that, in a manner analogous to breast cancer, estrogen might stimulate tumor growth in that population. Therapy consisted of diethylstilbesterol, (DES), 5 mg p.o. t.i.d., for a minimum of 6 weeks or until disease progression was noted.

The characteristics of patients on this study are shown in Table 1. Of the 24 patients entered and evaluable, 21 were males and 3 females. The median age was 37 with a range of 17 to 62 years. Five patients had disease limited to soft tissue plus lymph nodes while 19 patients had visceral metastases. Eighteen patients had received prior chemotherapy with DTIC or MeCCNU while nine patients received immunotherapy with BCG or DNCB. The median Karnofsky rating at entry on the study was 80 with a range of 50 to 100, implying that most patients were ambulatory. The distribution of steroid receptors in the melanoma patients treated with DES was as follows: estrogen receptor activity was detected in 5 of 24 (21%), progesterone in 8 of 22 (36%), and androgen in 1 of 20 (5%).

Two patients have had partial objective responses, one patient had disease stabilization, and 21 patients had progressive disease. The first partial responder was a 54-year-old white male who had progressive disease following treatment with BCG, high dose methotrexate, and MeCCNU. Metastatic melanoma was present in the soft tissues, lymph nodes, and spleen. Receptor analyses for estrogen, progesterone, and androgen were all negative. This patient had a greater than 90% partial response to DES that lasted for 7 months. The second partial responder was a 43-year-old white male who had progressive disease following treatment with MeCCNU. There was no detectable estrogen receptor in a biopsy of a lymph node metastasis. The patient received radiation therapy to a right axillary mass. A lung nodule in the left lower lobe disappeared on DES therapy for 4 months. A 28-year-old white male had disease stabilization. He had been previously treated with DTIC and MeCCNU. Melanoma was present in soft tissues and lymph nodes. Estrogen and androgen receptor activity was absent but a progesterone receptor was present. This patient had stable disease on DES for 6 months. Toxicity in this trial was minimal and consisted of minimal nausea, vomiting, and breast tenderness in males. No patients ceased treatment with DES because of toxicity.

It is of note that neither of the two responding patients had detectable estrogen receptors. Since the presence of estrogen receptor activity appears necessary but not sufficient for a direct biologic effect of the hormone on any target tissue, these results suggest that the DES-induced tumor regressions may have been mediated via an indirect mechanism of action — possibly by DES suppression of another hormone. Studies are currently in progress to evaluate this possibility. Since only five patients with detectable estrogen receptors have entered the trial, we cannot at this time determine the response rate of the melanoma patients who have estrogen receptors. Likewise since only three female patients have been treated with DES, the response rate in the female patients to estrogen therapy cannot be determined at this time.

Didolkar et al. have recently reported a trial of estramustine phosphate (estradiol conjugated with nitrogen mustard) in advanced malignant melanoma.[23] They reported a 20% objective response rate in 20 patients refractory to DTIC. Estrogen receptors were not determined so that no correlation between clinical response and receptor activity can be made.

V. CONCLUSIONS

The natural history of malignant melanoma suggests that hormones may influence the induction or growth of this tumor. Melanoma is rare before puberty with the incidence in females rising to a maximum in the childbearing years and again in the postmenopausal years. Rapid dissemination has been reported with pregnancy as well as spontaneous regressions postpartum. Regardless of stage or treatment, survival of female patients exceeds that of males. Objective tumor responses have been occasionally reported following various hormone manipulations. High-affinity, limited-capacity cytoplasmic receptors for estrogen binding have now been described for a significant number of patients with malignant melanoma. To date these steroid hormone receptors have not correlated with clinical aspects of this disease. A recent study has demonstrated objective tumor reponse following therapy with diethylstilbesterol in 0 of 5 estrogen-receptor positive and 2 of 19 estrogen-receptor negative patients. Further investigation is necessary to determine the biologic significance of steroid hormone receptors in melanoma and the mechanism of action of diethylstilbesterol in estrogen-receptor negative patients.

REFERENCES

1. **Luce, J. K., McBride, C. M., and Frei, E.,** Melanoma, in *Cancer Medicine,* Holland, J. F. and Frei, E., Eds., Lea and Febiger, Philadelphia, 1973, chap. 29.
2. **Gutterman, J. U., Mavigit, G., Reed., R., Richman, S., McBride, C. E., and Hersh, E. M.,** Immunology and immunotherapy of human malignant melanoma; historical review and perspectives for the future, *Semin. Oncol.,* 2, 155, 1975.
3. **Everson, T. C. and Cole, W. H.,** *Spontaneous Regression in Cancer,* W. B. Saunders, Philadelphia, 1966, 1.
4. **Bodenham, D. C. and Hale, B.,** Malignant melanoma, in *Endocrine Therapy in Malignant Disease,* Stoll, B. A., Ed., W. B. Saunders, Philadelphia, 1972, 377.
5. **McGovern, V. J.,** The classification of melanoma and its relationship with prognosis, *Pathology,* 2, 85, 1970.
6. **Pack, G. T. and Scharnagel, I. M.,** The prognosis for malignant melanoma in the pregnant woman, *Cancer (Philadelphia),* 4, 324, 1951.
7. **Nathanson, L., Hall, T. C., and Farber, S.,** Biological aspects of human malignant melanoma, *Cancer (Philadelphia),* 20, 650, 1967.
8. **White, L. P.,** Studies on melanoma, *N. Engl. J. Med.,* 260, 789, 1955.
9. **Conybeare, R. C.,** Malignant melanoma and pregnancy, *Obstet. Gynecol.,* 24, 451, 1964.

10. **Allen, E. P.,** Malignant melanoma, *Br. Med. J.,* 2, 1067, 1955.
11. **Byrd B. and McGanity, W. J.,** The effect of pregnancy on the clinical course of malignant melanoma, *South. Med. J.,* 47, 196, 1954.
12. **George, P. A., Fortner, J. G., and Pack, G. T.,** Melanoma with pregnancy, *Cancer (Philadelphia),* 13, 854, 1960.
13. **White, L. P., Linden, G., Breslow, L., and Harzfield, L.,** Studies on melanoma, *JAMA,* 177, 51, 1961.
14. **Shiu, M. H., Schottenfeld, D., Maclean, B., and Fortner, J. G.,** Adverse effect of pregnancy on melanoma, *Cancer (Philadelphia),* 37, 181, 1976.
15. **Johnson, R. O., Bisel, H., Andrews, N., Wilson, W., Rochlin, D., Segaloff, A., Krementz, E., Aust, J., and Ansfield, F.,** Phase I clinical study of 6 αmethylpregnene trione, *Cancer Chemother. Rep.,* 50, 671, 1966.
16. **Howes, W. E.,** Removal of testes in treatment of melanoma, *JAMA,* 123, 304, 1943.
17. **Meyer, H. W. and Gumport, S. L.,** Malignant melanoma, *Ann. Surg.,* 138, 643, 1953.
18. **Fisher, R. I., Neifeld, J. P., and Lippman, M. E.,** Estrogen receptors in human malignant melanoma, *Lancet,* 2, 337, 1976.
19. **Lippman, M. E. and Huff, K.,** Demonstration of androgen and estrogen receptors in human breast cancer using a new protamine sulfate assay, *Cancer (Philadelphia),* 38, 868, 1976.
20. **McGuire, W. L. and De LaGarza, M.,** Similarity of estrogen receptor in human and rat mammary carcinoma, *J. Clin. Endocrinol. Metab.,* 36, 548, 1973.
21. **Scatchard, G.,** Attractions of proteins for small molecules and ions, *Ann. N. Y. Acad. Sci.,* 51, 660, 1949.
22. **Fisher, R. I., Young, R. C., and Lippman, M. E.,** Diethylstilbesterol therapy of surgically non-resectable malignant melanoma, in *Proc. Am. Soc. Clin. Onco.,* Williams and Wilkins, Baltimore, 1976, 339.
23. **Didalkar, M. S., Catane, R., Lopez, R., and Holyoke, E. D.,** Estramustine phosphate in advanced malignant melanoma resistant to DTIC treatment, in *Proc. Am. Soc. Clin. Oncol.,* Williams and Wilkins, Baltimore, 1976, 381.

Chapter 5

THE ECTOPIC PRODUCTION OF HORMONES BY TUMORS

David P. Rose

TABLE OF CONTENTS

I. SOME GENERAL CONSIDERATIONS

A. Definition

The term "ectopic hormone production" was introduced by Liddle et al.[1] to describe the situation in which tumors of nonendocrine origin synthesize hormones, or substances which behave like a normal hormone; it may be expanded to include the secretion by endocrine gland tumors of hormones which are not physiologically associated with that gland. With this definition, we exclude calcitonin production by a medullary carcinoma of the thyroid, and β-human chorionic gonadotropin by a trophoblastic tumor, for example, because these hormones are secreted by the corresponding normal tissues.

In addition to the significance which the ectopic production of hormones has in understanding the mechanisms of carcinogenesis, it is an important aspect of neoplastic disease for two reasons. First, there is the need to recognize that an endocrinopathy, which may be the presenting feature, is due to an underlying neoplasm. Second, the presence of ectopically produced hormones in plasma or urine may provide a marker of tumor activity. This latter aspect is discussed in depth by Tormey and his colleagues in Volume II, Chapter 6.

B. Criteria for the Identification of Ectopic Hormone Production

Rees[2] has discussed the criteria which may be applied in order to establish the presence of ectopic hormone secretion, and stressed the inadequacy of merely showing increased hormonal activity in the presence of a tumor. These criteria include a fall in hormone level and regression of the clinical syndrome after removal of the tumor, the persistence of elevated hormone levels after removal of the gland which normally secretes that hormone, the demonstration of a difference in hormone concentration between the arterial and venous blood flow across the tumor, the presence of the hormone under consideration in tumor tissue, and the secretion of hormone by the tumor when it is cultured in vitro.

There are problems in applying each of these criteria. A reversal of the hormonal abnormality after tumor resection could occur, because the presence of the neoplasm is stimulating the gland which normally secretes the hormone. For example, Lewis and Deshpande[3] reported increased cortisol production rates in patients with advanced breast cancer which declined after hypophysectomy. Clearly, in this situation, the increased secretion of corticosteroids, the elevated plasma cortisol levels, and urinary 17-hydroxycorticosteroid excretions which may result arise from an effect of the tumor on pituitary function and not ectopic ACTH production.

There are few occasions when ectopic hormone production justifies ablation of the corresponding endocrine gland. Persistent elevations in hormone levels after endocrine surgery, providing support for the diagnosis of an ectopic hormone syndrome, have been described in cases of ectopic ACTH[4] and parathyroid hormone[5] production and the inappropriate secretion of antidiuretic hormone.[6]

The presence of a higher hormone concentration in the venous drainage of a tumor compared with its arterial inflow strongly supports the presence of ectopic hormone production. Unfortunately, this approach is often not possible because of anatomical or surgical difficulties. It has been used successfully in cases of ectopic gonadotropin,[7] ACTH and β-MSH,[8] parathyroid hormone,[9] and calcitonin[10] production.

At first sight, it might appear that the demonstration of a hormone in tumor tissue is firm evidence of ectopic synthesis. But, Unger et al.[11] have suggested that tumors adsorb hormones from the circulation (the "sponge" hypothesis), and there is some experimental evidence for such a phenomenon. The explanation may be that hormone polypeptides are taken up by receptors on the tumor surface; growth hormone, prolactin, and insulin membrane receptors have been demonstrated in some breast cancers,[12] for example.

Until recently, the demonstration of hormone secretion by the tumor in vitro has been hampered by the many problems associated with tissue culture of human cancers. Examples where this has been achieved include cases of a parathyroid hormone-secreting hepatoblastoma,[13] a renal-cell carcinoma which produced prolactin,[14] and calcitonin-secreting carcinomas of the breast[15] and bronchus.[16] Rees et al.[17] described an oat-cell carcinoma of the bronchus which produced eight different hormones, but only the secretion of ACTH and vasopressin were demonstrable in long-term tissue culture.

C. Hypotheses Regarding the Biological Basis for Ectopic Hormone Production

1. The Derepression Hypothesis

The basis of the derepression hypothesis is that differentiated somatic cells contain the genetic information of all potential cell phenotypes in the body, and that this may be retained in a latent (repressed) state. The concept has emerged that, as part of the process of neoplastic transformation, random derepression of DNA can occur. Should this happen to include the producer gene for a particular hormone, ectopic hormone production by the tumor would result.

The hormones secreted ectopically are all polypeptides; no cases have ever been reported involving, directly, the steroid or thyroid hormones. An explanation for this distinction is that peptide synthesis is genetically coded as a single step, so that only one alteration, derepression, is necessary for its initiation. Steroid hormone synthesis, on the other hand, involves a series of discrete steps, each catalyzed by a specific enzymic protein. In consequence, the chances of the appropriate, ectopically produced, enzymes for steroidogenesis all emerging together as part of the process of neoplastic transformation are infinitesimally small.

There is a wide variation between different tumors in the frequency with which they are responsible for ectopic hormone synthesis. At one extreme, carcinoma of the bronchus is the commonest tumor to be associated with the ectopic production of ACTH, MSH, vasopressin, parathyroid hormone, and, excluding the trophoblastic cancers, gonadotropins. In contrast, breast cancer is a rare cause of any clinically overt ectopic hormone syndrome, although some clones of breast carcinoma cells do secrete β-HCG,[18] and human placental lactogen,[19] and calcitonin.[15,20] Williams[21] has pointed out that such distinctions are not really compatible with a hypothesis of random derepression which, by chance, includes genes involved in polypeptide hormone production.

2. The Endocrine Cell Hypothesis

This is the most widely quoted, and probably the most favorably received, hypothesis at the present time. It is based on the concept that hormone-secreting cells are not confined to the endocrine glands as we conventionally think of them, but also occur in many other tissues. Under normal circumstances, these cells synthesize a restricted number of hormones, such as the catecholamines and 5-hydroxytryptamine. When neoplastic transformation takes place, they may continue to secrete the hormone appropriate to their anatomic site and cell type; for example, the secretion of 5-hydroxytryptamine by a carcinoid tumor derived from enterochromaffin cells. However, should a shift in gene function occur, perhaps because the genome for polypeptide synthesis is readily derepressed,[21] ectopic hormone production is initiated, and the carcinoid tumor then secretes, for example, ACTH.

One class of cells which could behave in this way is the APUD series described by Pearse and co-workers.[22,23] APUD is an acronym indicating that the cells of this group are characterized cytochemically by their amine content, amine precursor uptake, and capacity for decarboxylation of certain amino acids to yield amines.

The APUD cells are derived embryologically from the neural crest, from which they migrate to the primitive germ layers of the ectoderm. Neural crest migration of APUD cells throughout the primitive gut has been demonstrated, with particularly high concentrations occurring in the foregut.[24,25] When appropriately differentiated, their presence in structures derived from the primitive entoderm, such as the thyroid and parathyroid glands and the pancreatic islets, endows these organs with their endocrine function. Further, as the gastrointestinal tract is formed from the primitive entodermal canal, APUD cells are retained to become the primary source of the hormones released from the stomach, duodenum, and intestine.[26] In consequence, many of the known polypeptide-secreting cells, including the pituitary corticotrophs, have the same APUD characteristics as the chromaffin and argyrophil cells of the stomach and intestine and the Kultschitzky cells of the bronchial mucosa — cell types not known to synthesize polypeptides.

The endocrine APUD cell hypothesis provides an acceptable explanation for ACTH production by pancreatic islet cell tumors, and also by oat-cell carcinomas of the bronchus, if, as has been suggested, these latter arise from the Kultschitzky cells.[27] Where the hypothesis falters is when one considers the ectopic production of parathyroid hormone and gonadotropins; neither of these hormones are normally secreted by cells with the histochemical features of the APUD series. The APUD cell concept has been discussed in depth by Baylin[28] and Smith.[29]

3. Cell Hybridization

Warner[30] proposed that some ectopic hormone-secreting tumors arise from the fusion of neoplastic "nonendocrine" cells with endocrine cells, so that a mixed hormone-secreting phenotype is produced. Its intent is to cover those situations in which the APUD concept appears inappropriate, rather than to displace it, and to avoid consideration of the need for random derepression of the genome.

Table 1 gives the principal ectopic hormones that will be discussed in this review, the cancers with which they are most frequently associated, and the clinical manifestations with which they are usually associated.

TABLE 1

A Summary of the More Clinically Important Ectopically Produced Hormones to be Discussed in this Review

Hormone	Most frequently associated cancers	Clinical/metabolic manifestitations
ACTH (and CRF)	oat cell bronchial carcinoma	hypokalemic alkalosis
	thymoma	myopathy
	pancreatic tumors	
Vasopressin	bronchial carcinoma	dilutional hyponatremia
	papillary duodenal carcinoma	psychiatric disturbance
	pancreatic adenocarcinomas	convulsions, coma
Gonadotropins	(trophoblastic tumors)	precocious puberty
	bronchial carcinomas	gynecomastia
Parathyroid hormone	bronchial, usually squamous cell, carcinoma	hypercalcemia
	renal cell carcinoma	vomiting, constipation
	ovarian carcinoma	dehydration, coma
Insulin (and other hypoglycemic agents)	mesenchymal tumors	hypoglycemia
	bronchial carcinomas	
	adrenal carcinomas	
Erythropoietin	(renal-cell carcinoma)	erythrocytosis
	(benign renal lesions)	
	cerebellar hemangioblastoma	
	uterine fibromyomas	
	adrenocortical carcinomas	
	ovarian tumors, hepatomas	

Note: The diseases in parentheses are listed because, although they are not ectopic sources of the hormone, they are the most common tumors associated with that endocrinopathy.

II. ADRENOCORTICOTROPIC HORMONE AND CORTICOTROPIN-RELEASING FACTOR

Adrenocortical hyperfunction, due to ACTH stimulation, is responsible for the most common of ectopic hormone syndromes. The first recorded case was probably that described by Brown[31] in 1928. Although he did not associate the neoplasm with the endocrine abnormalities, his patient, a woman, had an oat-cell carcinoma of the bronchus, with bilateral adrenal hyperplasia, and the following typical features of Cushing's syndrome: trucal obesity, hirsutism, polycythemia, pigmentation, diabetes, and hypertension.

Since then, many cases of hyperadrenocorticism associated with a neoplasm other than that of the adrenals or pituitary gland have been reported in the literature. Liddle et al.[1] coined the term "ectopic ACTH" when describing five patients with tumors of nonendocrine origin, bilateral adrenal hyperplasia, and hypokalemia. Plasma ACTH levels were elevated, and corticotropic activity was demonstrated in both primary and metastatic tumor tissue.

Ectopic ACTH production with clinical manifestations is most frequently associated with carcinoma of the bronchus; these tumors, which are almost exclusively oat-cell carcinomas, account for approximately 50% of all cases.[32] The second most commonly associated tumors are thymic and pancreatic tumors (Table 2). In order to keep a true perspective of the situation, however, it should be noted that in a study by Kato et

TABLE 2

Neoplasms Associated with Ectopic ACTH Production

Tumor type	Approximate % of total cases
Carcinoma of the lung	50
Carcinoma of the thymus	10
Carcinoma of the pancreas[a]	10
Neoplasms of neural crest derivatives[b]	5
Medullary carcinoma of the thyroid	5
Bronchial adenoma (including carcinoid)	2
Miscellaneous	each < 2

[a]   Includes islet cell carcinomas and carcinoid.
[b]   Pheochromocytoma, neuroblastoma, paraganglioma and ganglioma

al.,[33] ectopic ACTH production was manifest clinically in only 2.8% of 138 patients with an oat-cell bronchial carcinoma, a figure close to the 2% estimated by Ross.[34]

A. Laboratory Investigations

1. Plasma and Tissue Ectopic ACTH

Early studies[32,35,36] and later experience[37] indicated that the immunological and physicochemical properties of the complete ectopic ACTH molecule are identical to those of the pituitary hormone. Recent investigations have shown that both ACTH fragments and "big" ACTH may occur in the tumor and plasma.

Pituitary ACTH consists of a single chain of 39 amino acids. The N-terminal fragment, amino acids 1-24, is the portion of the molecule responsible for steroidogenic activity; the C-terminal fragment, comprising amino acids 25-39, is biologically inert. Several groups have used specific antisera to demonstrate the presence of N-terminal and C-terminal fragments of ACTH in tumor extracts.[8,37-40] Orth et al.[37] employed three antisera directed against different parts of the ACTH molecule. A good correlation was demonstrated between bioactivity of ectopic ACTH in tumors and the N-terminal sequence 1-23 immunoreactivity. In addition, the tumors contained a peptide reacting immunologically with antibodies to N-terminal 1-13, but lacking biological activity, and also C-terminal 25-39 fragments.

A similar C-terminal fragment, composed of amino acids 18-39 was found in a bronchial carcinoid tumor extract.[8] Referred to as corticotropin-like intermediate lobe peptide (CLIP), it is absent from the human pituitary, but was originally isolated from the pars intermedia of rat and pig pituitaries.[41]

Big ACTH is an immunoreactive form of the hormone which is of considerably larger molecular weight than the 39 amino acid polypeptide, and lacks any significant steroidogenic activity.[42] Like big insulin, it is considered to be a prohormone; trypsinization in vitro converts big ACTH to the bioactive 39 amino acid polypeptide. Yalow et al.[43-45] found big ACTH in the tumor tissue and plasma from patients with ectopic ACTH production. In a study of 28 bronchial carcinoma patients without clinical evidence of hyperadrenocorticism, 14 of 15 primary tumors and all of 13 metastases contained immunoreactive ACTH, most of which was big ACTH; corresponding normal tissues showed no detectable hormone.[45] This high concentration of tumor big ACTH contrasts with that in extracts of normal pituitary glands, where the hormone is present largely as the 1-39 molecule.

One interesting feature of this investigation is that, histologically, the tumors were divided about equally between oat-cell carcinomas, adenocarcinomas, and squamous-cell carcinomas; yet, when ectopic ACTH production results in clinical disease, the tumor is nearly always of the oat-cell type. This suggests that only oat-cell carcinomas are likely to have a functioning enzymic mechanism for the conversion of big ACTH to the steroidogenic hormone.

In their study of ectopic ACTH production in carcinoma of the bronchus, Gewirtz and Yalow[45] also measured the afternoon plasma ACTH levels in 83 patients. Controls were patients with chronic obstructive pulmonary disease, other forms of lung disease, and healthy subjects. Just over half of the cancer patients and one third of those with chronic obstructive pulmonary disease had elevated plasma ACTH levels, the predominating component of which was big ACTH.

A recent study of ectopic ACTH by Bloomfield et al.[40] produced an interesting and provocative observation; it was found that *normal* lung tissue obtained from their patients contained ACTH at concentrations which correlated well with the amounts detected in the tumors themselves. The authors postulated that carcinoid and oat-cell tumors arise as foci of neoplastic change in a hyperactive field of endocrine cells, a proposal that is in keeping with the APUD cell hypothesis of ectopic hormone production discussed earlier.

2. Changes in Corticosteroid Levels

There have been a number of detailed studies of adrenal function in lung cancer patients unselected for any clinical features of Cushing's syndrome. McNamara et al.[46] studied 69 patients and, paradoxically, found more marked changes in the corticosteroid levels of those with epidermoid carcinomas than oat-cell carcinomas. Although the plasma cortisol levels were normal at 8 a.m., they were higher in the cancer patients than controls at 4 p.m. and 8 p.m., indicating a loss of the normal circadian rhythm. The 24-hr urinary 17-hydroxycorticosteroid excretion was elevated in the patients with epidermoid carcinomas, but not to a significant degree in those with oat-cell carcinomas.

Kawai et al.[47] devised a sequence of adrenocortical function tests for screening bronchial carcinoma patients for ectopic ACTH production. Included were plasma cortisol assays on blood samples obtained at 9 a.m. and 6 p.m. and the ratio of one to the other, urinary total 17-hydroxycorticosteroid and free cortisol excretions, a 1 mg dexamethasone suppression test, and a stimulation test with β^{1-24} ACTH (Synacten®). Only 9 of 23 lung cancer patients had normal results for all of the seven tests; abnormalities were detected most frequently in the dexamethasone suppression test (8 patients), the diurnal variation in plasma cortisol (7 patients), and the urinary free cortisol excretion (7 patients).

Imura et al.[48] have summarized their experience of 30 patients with tumors in which they demonstrated ACTH-like activity. There were 10 oat-cell carcinomas of the bronchus, nine other types of lung tumors including two carcinoids, four thymomas, and seven miscellaneous cancers. Seven patients had classical clinical signs of Cushing's syndrome, but none of these were cases of oat-cell bronchial carcinoma. Various tests of adrenal function were employed; 80% of patients had abnormalities, the most common being an elevated morning plasma cortisol, with loss of diurnal rhythm, and increased total urinary 17-hydroxycorticosteroid excretion.

3. Clinical Manifestations of the Ectopic ACTH Syndrome

Although the case of oat-cell carcinoma of the bronchus described by Brown[31] had many of the stigmata of Cushing's syndrome, this is unusual. It requires months or years of exposure to excessive cortisol stimulation to produce such abnormalities as truncal obesity, cutaneous striae, and osteoporosis. However, ectopic ACTH syn-

TABLE 3

Contrasting Clinical Features of the Ectopic ACTH Syndrome and Nonmalignant Cushing's Syndrome

	Ectopic ACTH syndrome	Nonmalignant Cushing's syndrome
Sex incidence	males	females
Age incidence	usually aged over 45 years	even distribution, 20 to 60 years
Rate of onset	acute	history usually over 1 year duration
Major symptoms and signs	muscle weakness, peripheral edema, weight loss, hypertension, impaired glucose tolerance, thirst, polyuria	truncal obesity, striae, plethora, hypertension, osteoporosis, hirsutism
Hypokalemic alkalosis	common	rare

drome is of acute onset, and is most frequently associated with rapid clinical deterioration, terminating in death after an average period of about 3 months.[49]

The major points which distinguish the ectopic ACTH syndrome from nonmalignant Cushing's syndrome are summarized in Table 3. The most common features are hypokalemic alkalosis, muscle weakness, hypertension, and impaired glucose tolerance. Hypokalemia is much more common in the ectopic ACTH syndrome, because the extremely high cortisol levels promote heavy renal losses of potassium.[49,50] Indeed, this abnormality is so striking that ectopic ACTH production should always be suspected in a patient who presents with Cushing's syndrome and hypokalemic alkalosis.

Extremely high cortisol and adrenal androgen production rates are reflected in the increased plasma cortisol, absence of circadian rhythm, and the markedly elevated urinary 17-hydroxycorticosteroids and 17-ketosteroids. All of these are more prominent in the ectopic ACTH syndrome than in nonmalignant Cushing's syndrome; in the latter, 17-ketosteroid excretion is normal or only slightly increased.

Further support for a diagnosis of ectopic ACTH syndrome is provided by failure to suppress steroidogenesis with dexamethasone, and the finding of elevated plasma ACTH levels. In one evaluation of the dexamethasone suppression test,[32] a dose of 8 mg/day for 2 days almost always decreased the urinary 17-hydroxycorticosteroid excretion by 40% or more in patients with excessive pituitary ACTH secretion. Primary adrenal tumors were unaffected by the exogenous corticosteroid, and in hypercorticosteroidism due to ectopic ACTH production, only 6% of the cases exhibited adrenal suppression. Failure to obtain suppression with dexamethasone because of ectopic ACTH production is readily distinguishable from autonomous cortisol secretion by a primary adrenal tumor, because in the former case, the plasma ACTH is elevated, and in the latter instance, it is undetectable.

4. Ectopic Production of Corticotropin-Releasing Factor

When dexamethasone does cause suppression of cortisol secretion in a case of apparent ectopic ACTH syndrome, the probable explanation is that the tumor is, in fact, producing a corticotropin-releasing factor (CRF).

Upton and Amatruda[51] first reported the presence of CRF in tumors from four patients with what appeared to be ectopic ACTH syndrome: two with oat-cell carcinomas of the bronchus and two with pancreatic cancers. All showed suppression of cortisol secretion by dexamethasone.

A similar case of ectopic CRF production by a medullary carcinoma of the thyroid was described by Birkenhäger et al.[52] In this patient, there was a significant arteriovenous difference in CRF activity across the thyroid gland, and CRF was demonstrated in the tumor tissue. An additional diagnostic point in favor of ectopic CRF being

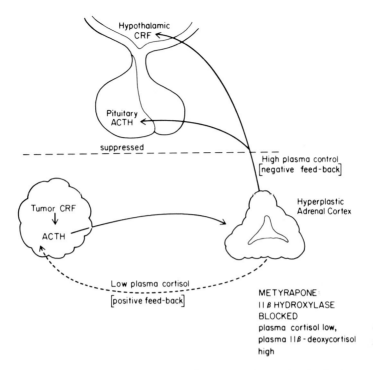

FIGURE 1.   The feedback regulation of ectopic corticotropin-releasing factor as proposed by Suda, T., Demura, H., Demura, R., Wakabayashi, I., Namura, K., Odagiri, E., and Shizume, K., Corticotropin-releasing factor-like activity in ACTH producing tumors, *J. Clin. Endocrinol. Metab.*, 44, 440, 1977.

responsible for the Cushing's syndrome was that the plasma cortisol increase after lysine vasopressin administration was similar to that seen in pituitary-dependent Cushing's syndrome; in the ectopic ACTH syndrome there is usually an absence of response.[53]

Tumors which show CRF activity frequently also produce ACTH.[52,54,55] In one study, 7 out of 11 tumors had significant CRF activity, and in 6 of them, ectopic ACTH was also demonstrated by both bioassay and radioimmunoassay.[54]

Suda et al.[55] have speculated that the ectopic secretion of CRF by tumors may not be autonomous, but subject to feed back regulation. Their patient had shown a response to metyrapone, and the tumor extract contained both ACTH and CRF activity. It was suggested that the tumor CRF could stimulate tumor ACTH secretion, and that regulatory feedback existed between tumor CRF and the circulating cortisol level. In this way, the reduction in plasma cortisol by metyrapone would be responsible for tumor CRF-stimulated release of tumor ACTH, and, so, adrenal steroidogenesis with an elevation in plasma 11-deoxycortisol. This fascinating concept is illustrated in Figure 1.

5. Treatment of Ectopic ACTH/CRF Syndrome

Because of its frequent association with bronchogenic carcinoma, the prognosis for most patients with the features of the ectopic ACTH syndrome is extremely poor. Occasionally, the tumor is amenable to complete surgical resection, in which case there is immediate reversal of the hyperadrenocorticism.[56] An alternative, in the rare patient with unresectable disease, but a tumor of low-grade malignancy, is bilateral adrenalectomy. "Medical adrenalectomy" has also been used successfully, by employing drugs which block cortisol synthesis. Metyrapone, which impairs 11β-hydroxylase activity, is an effective agent in some cases, although the doses which have to be employed may be very large.[32,57,58] Aminoglutethimide, a drug which blocks the conversion of cholesterol to pregnenolone, is also effective.[59]

III. MELANOCYTE-STIMULATING HORMONE

Ectopic melanocyte-stimulating hormone (MSH) production appears always to occur in association with that of ACTH.[17,60-64] Abe et al.[65] found that the biological activity of ectopic MSH is predominantly due to β-MSH, but, in addition, some stimulatory activity may be present which cannot be accounted for by either β- or α-MSH. This may represent N-terminal fragments of ACTH or the presence of β- and γ-lipotropic hormone (LPH), both of which have MSH biological activity, and react in immunoassay.[66] Bloomfield et al.[67] found that the elution pattern of major MSH-immunoreactivity on gel filtration of extracts of six ectopic ACTH-secreting tumors corresponded with that of β- and γ-LPH. In another patient, it was a peptide of larger molecular weight than ACTH.[68]

A current view is that the 22 amino acid peptide, referred to as β-MSH, does not, in fact, exist in man under normal circumstances,[66,69,70] but that which is detected by radioimmunoassay is a whole series of larger molecules, all of which contain the β-MSH sequence. A small β-MSH molecule which was identified in two ectopic ACTH-secreting tumors may have been formed from β-LPH by enzymatic degradation.[2]

The clinical features of ectopic MSH production are overshadowed in importance by those of ACTH-induced hypercorticosteroidism. When the circulating levels of MSH are high, stimulation of melanin formation by the melanocytes of skin and mucous membranes results in hyperpigmentation.

IV. VASOPRESSIN

In 1957, Schwartz et al.[71] described two patients with carcinoma of the bronchus, a syndrome of hyponatremia, persistently hyperosmotic urine, and failure to conserve sodium in the face of depletion. Although they recognized that the electrolyte imbalance was due to inappropriately high antidiuretic hormone (vasopressin, ADH) levels, it was suggested that the tumors were stimulating ADH secretion from the neurohypophysis. Later, Amatruda et al.[72] used a bioassay to demonstrate the presence of ADH-like activity in an extract of an oat-cell bronchial carcinoma removed from a patient with the syndrome of inappropriate ADH secretion.

Since that time, many reports of the syndrome have been published, almost always in association with oat-cell or anaplastic carcinoma of the bronchus. The few exceptions include a papillary carcinoma of the duodenum,[73] pancreatic adenocarcinomas,[74,75] bronchial carcinoids,[76] and cancer of the breast[75] and esophagus.[77] Other tumor sites have been recorded, but these involve the brain and the inappropriate antidiuresis may have been a consequence of intracranial damage rather than ectopic hormone production.

A. Tumor ADH

The peptide appears to be biologically, chemically, and immunologically indistinguishable from arginine vasopressin. Lipscombe et al.[78] showed that material with antidiuretic activity extracted from a bronchial carcinoma behaved in an identical manner to arginine (human) vasopressin on a Sephadex G-25® column, and was clearly distinguishable from lysine (porcine) vasopressin in a counter-current distribution system. In other studies, similar material was found to react with antibodies to arginine vasopressin[75,79] with loss of its biological activity.[75] Finally, tumor tissue from a patient with the inappropriate ADH secretion syndrome was shown, in vitro, to incorporate ^{3}H-labeled arginine into a peptide chemically similar to arginine vasopressin.[80]

Neurophysin is the collective name for a small group of polypeptides which act as carrier proteins for vasopressin and oxytocin.[81] The synthesis and secretion of neurophysin closely parallels those of the two hormones, and so it is of particular interest that these peptides have been identified in ADH-containing tumors.[17,76] The patient described by Rees et al.[17] presented with an oat-cell carcinoma of the bronchus and Cushing's syndrome due to ectopic ACTH production. Control of the hyperadrenocorticism with aminoglutethimide revealed inappropriate ADH secretion as reflected by hyponatremia. The tumor contained a remarkable collection of hormones: arginine vasopressin, oxytocin, neurophysin, ACTH, corticotropin-like intermediate lobe peptide, β-MSH, insulin, and prolactin.

B. Clinical Features

The clinical picture resulting from inappropriate ADH secretion is essentially that of water intoxication. If water retention is sufficient to cause the plasma sodium to fall below 120 meq/ℓ, headache, anorexia, nausea, and vomiting are likely to develop.[77] Neurological signs are common when a level is less than 115 meq/ℓ, with mental confusion, lassitude, extrapyramidal disturbances, and convulsions. Death occurs frequently when the plasma sodium concentration is reduced to below 100 meq/ℓ.

In addition to hyponatremia and plasma hypoosmolality, hypokalemia and hypocalcemia are common;[77] the only other finding on routine investigation is the excretion of small volumes of urine which is inappropriately concentrated for a patient with hypotonic extracellular fluid, and which contains large amounts of sodium relative to the hyponatremic state. Increased levels of ADH can be demonstrated in the urine[82] and plasma,[6,83] which are not suppressed by a water load. Some patients also have a proximal renal tubular defect, with glycosuria, generalized amino aciduria, and hypophosphatemia.[84-86]

C. Treatment

Because of its frequent association with oat-cell carcinoma of the bronchus, a permanent cure of the inappropriate ADH secretion syndrome is rarely possible. At least two cases have been reported in which surgical resection of a bronchogenic carcinoma led to a prompt remission of the hormonal defect.[79,87] In one instance, reappearance of the hyponatremic state preceded direct evidence of tumor recurrence.

Restriction of water intake to a level where urinary and insensible losses induce negative fluid balance (500 to 1000 mℓ) will correct the hyponatremia within a few days, and reverse the symptoms of water intoxication.[77,88] It is generally recommended that if the hyponatremia is life threatening (plasma sodium concentration of 100 to 115 meq/ℓ), not only should water intake be restricted, but hypertonic saline be given by infusion. However, in one recent series of cases, this was ineffective in all of eight patients so treated; in each instance it was followed by the prompt excretion of the infused sodium.[77] Hantmann et al.[89] have recommended, that in extreme cases, negative water balance be induced by intravenous frusemide, with monitoring of the urinary sodium and potassium losses and their replacement hourly during the diuresis.

V. GONADOTROPINS

The tumors which typically produce gonadotropins are the choriocarcinomas of placental, ovarian, and testicular origin, but the source of the hormone in these cases cannot be regarded as ectopic. Gonadotropin production by nontrophoblastic tumors has been reported most commonly in association with bronchogenic carcinomas[9,90-93] and hepatomas or hepatoblastomas in children.[94-97]

The ectopic gonadotropin syndrome of childhood is characterized by precocious puberty, with premature development of secondary sex characteristics, advanced skeletal maturation, and hyperplasia of prostatic and testicular interstitial cells.[98] These changes are all attributable to activity of an LH-like peptide; no case of ectopic gonadotropin production in childhood has involved FSH, and so, because LH in the absence of FSH has no apparent effect in girls, the clinical syndrome occurs only in boys.

The clinical manifestation of ectopic gonadotropin production in lung cancer is gynecomastia;[9,92] testicular biopsy reveals interstitial cell hyperplasia.[90] Both Fusco and Rosen[90] and Faiman et al.[7] commented on the histological features of the tumors in their cases of bronchogenic carcinomas with gynecomastia; both were epidermoid cancers and were composed of sheets of large cells with vesicular cytoplasm and a tendency to form a follicular pattern. Cottrell et al.,[93] on the other hand, reported four cases which represented a broad spectrum of histological types.

In 1969, Rosen and Weintraub[99] pointed out that none of the reports of ectopic gonadotropin production published up until that time permitted a distinction between LH and HCG as the involved peptide. Later, they demonstrated the presence of an HCG-like peptide in nontrophoblastic tumors,[100] and the production of HCG in vitro by a cell line derived from an undifferentiated bronchial carcinoma.[101] Three cell clones were derived from this tumor, each of which showed differing rates of synthesis and secretion of HCG and its α and β sub units.[102]

There has been just one report of an FSH-secreting carcinoma of the bronchus.[7] In this case, the patient had an adenocarcinoma with gynecomastia and hypertrophic pulmonary osteoarthropathy; radioimmunoassays demonstrated elevated plasma FSH and LH, with a higher concentration of FSH (but not LH) in pulmonary venous than in arterial blood. Both the clinical and hormonal abnormalities were reversed after pneumonectomy. Immunoreactive FSH and LH were demonstrated in the tumor tissue.

VI. PARATHYROID HORMONE: PROSTAGLANDINS

Hypercalcemia in the cancer patient is usually associated with osteolytic metastases, but it may also occur in their absence. Some of these cases are the result of the ectopic production of a parathyroid hormone (PTH)-like peptide. The first description appeared in the published case records of the Massachusetts General Hospital.[103] During the discussion of a patient with a renal-cell carcinoma and hyperparathyroidism, Albright suggested that the syndrome was due to the elaboration of PTH, or a substance of similar biological activity, by the tumor. Similar cases were reported later;[104,105] in three patients described by Plimpton and Gellhorn,[105] the tumors were operable, and their removal produced a prompt fall in the serum calcium.

A. Tumor Types Associated with Ectopic PTH Production

A wide variety of tumors have been associated with hypercalcemia, attributable to ectopic production of PTH or a PTH-like peptide. Omenn et al.[106] reviewed 64 cases and added 9 of their own. In 30 cases, treatment of the tumor reversed the hyperparathyroid state, normal serum calcium levels being attained within 48 hr. The most frequent tumor sites were kidney (21), lung (20), ovary (6), and pancreas (5). It is noteworthy that 13 of the 20 lung tumors were squamous-cell carcinomas, and only 1 was an oat-cell carcinoma; the histological type was unspecified in the other six. This contrasts with the situation in ectopic ACTH syndrome due to lung cancers, where the predominant tumor is the oat-cell carcinoma.

Rosen and Weintraub[107] reported a case of gastric carcinoid without bone involvement, in which there was hypercalcemia and PTH-like activity in the tumor. This tumor also contained calcitonin, and was producing alpha subunits of the glycoprotein hormones. The syndrome is rare in childhood cancers; only two reports appear to have been published. The first of these was a 2-year-old boy with a hepatoblastoma,[13] and the other, investigated in much less detail, was a 7-year-old boy with anaplastic carcinoma of the testis.[98]

B. Demonstration of the Ectopic PTH-like Peptide

PTH-like peptides have been demonstrated in extracts of various tumors, including renal-cell carcinomas,[9,108] squamous-cell bronchial carcinomas,[109,110] hepatoma,[111] and breast cancers.[112,113]

Tashjian et al.[108] studied six cancer patients with hyperparathyroidism believed to be of ectopic origin, and seven other patients with malignant disease not associated with hypercalcemia. The tumors, but not control normal tissue, from the six patients with suspected ectopic PTH syndrome all contained a material which reacted with antibovine PTH antisera. This was not detected in the other seven tumors. Later, these workers obtained supporting evidence for their conclusion that the tumors contained PTH, or a peptide very much like it, when they showed that extracts specifically inhibited the direct complement fixation by purified bovine PTH and rabbit antibovine PTH antibody.[114]

Sherwood et al.[110] used a radioimmunoassay to measure PTH-like activity in extracts of tumors from 13 patients with hypercalcemia; significant levels were found in seven. On ultracentrifugation, this material also sedimented in a sucrose gradient as a single entity, with a molecular size similar to human or bovine PTH. One patient, in whom hyperparathyroidism was subsequently excluded at autopsy, had increased PTH in the plasma.

Supporting evidence for the ectopic production of PTH by tumors has also been provided by arteriovenous gradient measurements and studies of tumor tissue in vitro. By radioimmunoassay techniques, Buckle et al.[9] were able to demonstrate the presence of an arteriovenous gradient of PTH across a kidney bearing an adenocarcinoma. The PTH concentration in renal arterial blood was only 0.65 ng/mℓ, but in venous blood draining the tumor it was 2.55 ng/mℓ. Tashjian[13] obtained tumor cells from the ascitic fluid of a child with a hepatoblastoma, hypercalcemia, and hypophosphatemia. In culture, these cells secreted immunoreactive PTH. Two reports of PTH-like material in breast cancer tissue[112,113] are of special interest, because these tumors have not otherwise been associated with ectopic PTH production.

Several investigators have demonstrated that there are immunoreactive differences between parathyroid gland-secreted PTH and the hormone produced ectopically by tumors. These differences result in a variation in the ratio of immunologic to biologic activity. Riggs et al.[115] were able to distinguish between immunoreactive PTH in the serum of patients with primary hyperparathyroidism and ectopic hyperparathyroidism. Using an antiserum directed against the C-terminal fragments, the serum immunoreactive PTH was high in the cases of primary parathyroid disease, and there was a good correlation between it and the serum calcium level. In ectopic hyperparathyroidism, it frequently was not possible to detect PTH at all with this antiserum, and yet the serum calcium concentrations were very high. One explanation is that tumor cells may produce a PTH precursor, but lack the ability to convert it to the form in which PTH is normally secreted from the parathyroid glands.[115] This would involve enzymic cleavage to give the biologically inactive C-terminal fragment and the biologically active N-terminal fragment.

Benson et al.[116] also observed differences in the PTH species which circulate in ectopic hyperparathyroidism and primary hyperparathyroidism. Three peaks of PTH-like immunoreactivity emerged when plasmas from patients with either disease were passed through Bio-Gel P-150® columns. But, in three of the six patients with the ectopic syndrome, there was a strikingly increased amount of a high molecular weight component which eluted in advance of both proPTH and native PTH. Rees[2] has suggested that this is the preproPTH described by Kemper et al.[117]

C. Clinical Features

The clinical picture of the ectopic PTH syndrome arises exclusively from the hypercalcemia; anorexia, weight loss, nausea, thirst, constipation, lethargy, and mental confusion proceed in severe cases to intractable vomiting, dehydration, azotemia, and coma. Inability to produce a concentrated urine results in polyuria.

In making the clinical distinction between hypercalcemia due to primary hyperparathyroidism and ectopic PTH production, Lafferty[118] stressed the following features as favoring the latter diagnosis: a male with recent weight loss, who is anemic, with a serum calcium concentration of more than 14 mg/100 mℓ, and a serum chloride of less than 102 meq/ℓ. Renal calculi and bone resorption are almost never seen as clinical sequelae of ectopic PTH production. Other features to bear in mind when considering the differential diagnosis are that the serum phosphorus is reduced in ectopic PTH syndrome, as it is in primary hyperparathyroidism, but elevated in hypercalcemia due to bone metastases, and that the serum calcium concentration is not influenced by corticosteroid therapy.

D. Treatment

Removal of the tumor which is the ectopic source of PTH will produce a prompt reversal of symptoms due to hypercalcemia. When this is not possible, control of the hypercalcemia may be achieved by medical means. The simplest course is to increase the renal solute load with intravenous saline. Alternatives include the use of sodium sulfate infusions and treatment with chelating agents, calcitonin or mithramycin.[119]

E. Prostaglandin Production by Tumors

Because only a minority of hypercalcemic cancer patients without bone metastases show ectopic production of PTH, or PTH-like substances, a search has been made for other calcium-mobilizing agents.

The prostaglandins (PG) are cyclic fatty acids with a wide range of biological activities. They are all composed of a 20 carbon carboxylic acid containing a cyclopentane ring; structural modifications endow each compound with its specific function(s).

Prostaglandins of the E series (PGE, Figure 2) are potent stimulators of bone resorption in vitro,[120] and PGE_2 has been shown to cause hypercalcemia in animal tumor models.[121-123] Powell et al.[124] found that tumor tissue extracts from patients with hypercalcemia, but normal serum PTH levels, induced bone resorption in vitro, and one possibility which they considered was that these neoplasms were secreting prostaglandins.

Indomethacin and aspirin, two inhibitors of prostaglandin synthetase, suppress the

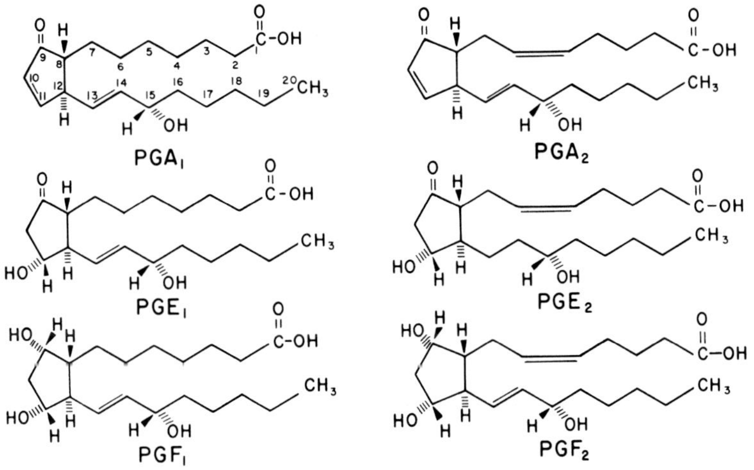

FIGURE 2.   Structural relationship of the prostaglandins.

osteolytic activity in vitro of some human breast cancers[125] and the development of bone metastases in rats[125] and rabbits.[126] Brereton et al.[127] demonstrated PG-like activity in tumor tissue from a hypercalcemic patient and a reduction in the serum calcium concentration after treatment with prostaglandin inhibitors. Further studies have confirmed the presence of PGE in some tumor tissues[128,129] and its production by human renal-cell carcinoma cells in culture.[130]

The principal urinary metabolite of prostaglandin E_1 and E_2 is 7α-hydroxy-5,11-diketotetranorprostane-1,16-dioic acid; its excretion is elevated in cancer patients with hypercalcemia, but normal plasma PTH levels.[131] When prostaglandin synthesis was inhibited by aspirin or indomethacin, the urinary excretion of the metabolite and of calcium and the plasma calcium concentration were all reduced.

This work is potentially of considerable clinical importance. Powles et al.[132] tested 38 breast cancers for in vitro osteolysis. Of 15 patients whose tumors did not show osteolytic activity, none had bone metastases when tested, and none were detected over a 3-year follow-up period. Tumors from the other 23 patients were active; 4 had bone metastases when first tested, and 3 later developed metastatic bone disease. The osteolytic activity in eight of nine tumors examined showed reduced osteolysis in vitro when incubated with a prostaglandin inhibitor.

It has been suggested that the capacity of tumors to synthesize prostaglandins is related to the likelihood of their metastasizing to bone.[133,134] Bennett et al.[134] found more prostaglandin-like material in breast cancers than in benign tumors or normal breast tissue. Cancers from patients with bone metastases synthesized more PG in vitro than did those with negative bone scans. Curiously, however, prostaglandins of the F series, the osteolytic activity of which is in dispute, correlated best with the presence or absence of bone metastases. It remains to be seen whether treatment with inhibitors of PG synthesis will reduce the risk of metastases to bone.

VII. INSULIN AND OTHER HYPOGLYCEMIC FACTORS

Hypoglycemia has been described as a complication of a variety of nonpancreatic islet cell tumors. In approximately two thirds of cases, these patients have large mensenchymal tumors, including fibrosarcomas, neurofibromas, neurofibrosarcomas, mesotheliomas, rhabdomyosarcomas, leiomyosarcomas, and lymphosarcomas. Primary hepatic tumors account for about 20% of cases.[135] In one series of 100 cases occurring in adults, all of these tumors weighed between 800 and 10,000 g, with an average weight of 2000 g.[135]

A. Mechanism for the Hypoglycemia

1. Ectopic Insulin Production

Synthesis of insulin by the tumor is not a common cause of hypoglycemia associated with nonpancreatic tumors, but it is the one that is most clearly attributable to ectopic hormone production. Immunoreactive insulin has been detected in fibrosarcomas,[136] leiomyosarcomas,[137] hemangiopericytomas,[138] carcinoma of the bronchus,[136] bronchial carcinoid tumor,[139] and carcinoma of the cervix.[140] It has been questioned whether the small amounts of insulin detected in these tumor tissues could be solely responsible for hypoglycemia,[137,138] but this might be explained by a continuous discharge of hormone into the circulation.

Unger et al.[11] performed studies to characterize the immunoreactive insulin-like material which they found in extracts of a metastatic bronchogenic carcinoma. Like insulin, it was inactivated by treatment with cysteine, which disrupts the disulfide bridges in the molecule, and it showed identical behavior to insulin on cellulose acetate electrophoresis. The concentration of the presumed ectopically produced insulin in the metastasis was 260 mU/g, which gave a total tumor content of approximately 260 U. Despite this high concentration relative to that in tumors from hypoglycemic patients reported by others,[138] there were no indications of hypoglycemia in this case. However, the tumor also contained glucagon, whose potency as a hyperglycemic agent, on a molar basis, far exceeds that of insulin to induce hypoglycemia.

2. Nonsuppressible Insulin-like Activity

Doubts that ectopic insulin production is an important factor in many of the cases of hypoglycemia associated with nonendocrine tumors have stimulated the pursuit of alternative explanations. Insulin-like biological activity in normal plasma is due to a number of components other than insulin itself, the best characterized being nonsuppressible insulin-like activity stemming from an acetic acid, ethanol-soluble peptide (NSILA-s). NSILA-s has a molecular weight of 7400, it behaves biologically like insulin in vitro and in vivo, but it does not react with antiinsulin antibodies.

Megyesi et al.[141] employed a specific radioreceptor assay to demonstrate elevated levels of NSILA-s in the plasma of five patients with hypoglycemia complicating nonpancreatic tumors. Two other patients with hypoglycemia associated with breast cancer and reticulum-cell sarcoma, respectively, had normal plasma NSILA-s concentrations, as did patients with hepatoma, fibrosarcoma, or carcinoma of the bronchus *without* hypoglycemia.

3. Increased Glucose Consumption by Tumor

Several authors have suggested that excessive glucose utilization by the tumor may be responsible for hypoglycemia.[137,138,142,143] Certainly, the tremendous size of many of these neoplasms, and the finding of high tumor glycogen content in the face of hypoglycemia in the host,[142] give support to this possibility. There have been attempts to assess the arteriovenous glucose-concentration gradient across the tumor, but the observed differences were negligible, and did not provide any convincing evidence of preferential glucose uptake by the tumor.[144,145] There is an animal model for tumor-related hypoglycemia, but studies with ^{14}C-labeled glucose failed to demonstrate excessive glucose utilization by the neoplasm.[146]

B. Clinical Features

The diagnosis should be considered in any patient with a nonpancreatic tumor who meets Whipple's triad of criteria for organic hypoglycemia: (1) symptoms of hypoglycemia in the fasting state, (2) blood glucose less than 50 mg/100 mℓ during an attack, and (3) relief of symptoms in response to intravenous glucose. Usually in these cases there is a slow fall in the blood glucose, and the hypoglycemia is prolonged. The principal symptoms arise from subacute neuroglycopenia: headache, impaired visual acuity, and mental confusion, together with various behavioral changes and neurological signs.

Laboratory investigation confirms the presence of hypoglycemia, and the appropriate tests exclude adrenal, pituitary, and hepatic insufficiency as the alternative mechanisms. Glucose tolerance tests typically give results which are similar to those sometimes seen in cases of insulinoma; there is a rapid increase in blood glucose, followed by a prompt return to normal or hypoglycemic levels.[142] The characteristic response of a patient with insulinoma to intravenous tolbutamide, a marked hypoglycemia which persists for 3 hr or longer, does not occur.

C. Treatment

When possible, surgical removal of the tumor will completely correct the symptoms. In inoperable cases, zinc glucagon and streptozotocin may be effective and are more likely to control the hypoglycemic episodes than glucocorticoids.

VIII. ERYTHROPOIETIN

Erythrocytosis due to excessive erythropoietin production has been described in association with a number of different neoplasms. If renal-cell carcinoma is excluded on the grounds that the kidney is the normal site of secretion, the most common responsible tumor is cerebellar hemangioblastoma, which accounts for approximately 20% of cases. Erythrocytosis is said to occur in 10 to 20% of patients with cerebellar hemangioblastomas,[135] but elevated plasma erythropoietin levels have been sought and demonstrated in relatively few cases. Indeed, until recently, the study of ectopic erythropoietin production was handicapped by lack of a satisfactory assay.[147]

Other neoplasms in which the production of erythropoietin-like material has been demonstrated by bioassay include fibromyomas of the uterus,[148-150] adrenocortical carcinomas,[151] virilizing tumors of the ovary,[151] hepatomas,[152] pheochromocytomas,[153] and Wilms' tumor.[154-156]

The studies by Wrigley et al.[149] are particularly valuable because, unlike earlier investigators, they employed a standard erythropoietin preparation in their bioassay. Erythropoietin activity was demonstrated in an extract of a uterine fibromyoma and in fluid from cysts which had formed within the tumor; removal of the tumor promptly corrected the erythrocytosis. Ossias et al.[150] also studied a case of uterine fibromyoma with erythrocytosis. Before surgery, elevated erythropoietin activity was detected in serum and urine. Tumor extracts contained erythropoietin-like activity which was abolished by antierythropoietin antisera.

The clinical feature of ectopic erythropoietin production is erythrocytosis. Unlike polycythemia vera, splenomegaly is not present, and the blood leukocyte and platelet counts are normal.

IX. ECTOPIC INTESTINAL HORMONES

A. Gastrin

Ectopic production of gastrin, which is normally secreted from the antral part of the stomach, arises typically from a nonbeta-cell tumor of the pancreas, as described originally by Zollinger and Ellison.[157] It has also been reported in association with tumors of the duodenum.[158]

The clinical syndrome is dominated by peptic ulceration, often occurring in the jejunum as well as the duodenum. Diarrhea may be a prominent symptom, perhaps because gastrin inhibits water and electrolyte intestinal absorption,[159] or as a result of the simultaneous ectopic production of vasoactive intestinal peptide.

Diagnosis may be confirmed by radioimmunoassay of serum gastrin levels.[160] Gastrin occurs in the blood in several forms; in the resting interdigestive period the principal component is a large molecule referred to as "big—big" gastrin.[161] Upon stimulation of gastrin secretion, three other forms appear in the circulation. Two are the heptadecapeptide amines described by Gregory and Tracy,[162] and the other is a larger, more basic molecule ("big" gastrin).[160]

In one study, the biologically active gastrin in an extract of a tumor from a patient with Zollinger-Ellison syndrome was the pair of heptadecapeptides.[163] Yalow and Berson[164] reported that sera from patients with Zollinger-Ellison syndrome contain up to 50% of immunoreactive gastrin as a heptapeptide ("little" gastrin), and the remainder, often the major portion, as "big" gastrin.

A pair of peptides of identical amino acid composition, but different charge, were isolated from Zollinger-Ellison tumor tissue.[165] These two peptides, which corresponded in their properties to "big" gastrin, contained the heptadecapeptide amine as a C-terminal sequence, linked to the remainder of the molecule by the peptide bond lysyl—glutaminyl. Both were highly active stimulators of gastric acid secretion. "Big—big" gastrin was found to comprise less than 2% of the immunoreactive gastrin in a Zollinger-Ellison tumor extract and plasma from patients with the syndrome.[161]

Rehfeld and Stadil[166] examined the gastrin content of sera from 15 patients with the Zollinger-Ellison syndrome by gel filtration. Immunoreactive gastrin emerged from the columns as four components; among these one corresponded to the two heptadecapeptides, one to big gastrin, and a third, a "mini" gastrin which was probably a tridecapeptide. No component was identified corresponding to "big—big" gastrin.

B. Vasoactive Intestinal Polypeptide

Vasoactive intestinal polypeptide (VIP), a 28 amino acid peptide structurally similar to secretin and glucagon, has a relaxant effect on gastric and gallbladder muscle, but a stimulating effect on intestinal muscle.[167,168] Bloom et al.[169] described five patients, four with carcinomas of the pancreas and one with a retroperitoneal ganglioneuroblastoma, who developed a syndrome of watery diarrhea, hypokalemia, and achlorhydria. All of these tumors contained radioimmunoassayable VIP, and high levels of the peptide were also detected in plasma samples; histochemical examination showed that they were composed of cells of the APUD series (see Section I.C.2). In another study, 13 patients with pancreatic islet cell adenoma, five with bronchial carcinoma, and one each with a pheochromocytoma or a ganglioblastoma, had the watery diarrhea syndrome and elevated plasma VIP concentrations. The pheochromocytoma, the ganglioblastoma, and the only bronchial carcinoma assayed, all contained large amounts of VIP.[170]

C. Gastric Inhibitory Peptide and Enteroglucagon

Gastric inhibitory peptide (GIP), an intestinal inhibitor of gastric secretion, has not been synthesized, but its chemical structure is known.[171] GIP and VIP may be considered as phylogenetic derivatives of the secretin—glucagon molecule; GIP shares 15 amino acid residues with glucagon, nine with secretin, and four with VIP.

Elias et al.[172] reported the case of a patient with a nonbeta-cell pancreatic tumor and the watery diarrhea syndrome described above. Histoimmunofluorescent examination of the tumor for GIP was strongly positive, and ectopic production of this hormone was considered to be responsible for the intestinal dysfunction; the tissue was not examined for VIP.

One case of an enteroglucagon-secreting neoplasm has been reported.[173] This patient had a renal tumor which histochemically fulfilled the critera for the APUD cell series, and histologically resembled a carcinoid or a pancreatic-islet α cell tumor. The clinical features were severe constipation, symptoms of intestinal malabsorption, confirmed by laboratory investigation, and intestinal changes characterized by villous hypertrophy. These abnormalities were all corrected by removal of the tumor. Later studies demonstrated the presence of a large amount of material with glucagon-like immunoreactivity in the tumor, which appeared to be identical with enteroglucagon.[174]

X. ECTOPIC THYROTROPIN

Four distinct substances have been isolated with thyrotropic activity: pituitary thyroid-stimulating hormone or thyrotropin (TSH), long-acting thyroid stimulators (LATS), human chorionic thyrotropin (HCT), and molar thyroid-stimulating hormone (M-TSH).

HCT is a polypeptide secreted by the normal placenta. Although it has biological activity which is similar to that of human pituitary TSH,[175] its immunoreactivity is more akin to that of bovine and porcine TSH.[176,177]

M-TSH is secreted by trophoblastic tumors; it does not cross-react immunologically with human or bovine pituitary TSH, LATS, or HCT.[175,178] Inasmuch as gonadotropins have little or no thyrotropic activity,[179,180] and patients with choriocarcinoma do not become hyperthyroid in the presence of high HCG levels, M-TSH does not appear to be closely related structurally gonadotropins.

In 1960, Dowling et al.[179] reported the association of hydatidiform mole with clinical and biochemical evidence of hyperthyroidism; the abnormal thyroid function was corrected after evacuation of the uterus. Since that time, the complication has become well recognized.[181,182] A similar relationship has been described between embryonal tumors of the testes and hyperthyroidism.[183,184]

Odell et al.[182] reported their experience of 11 patients with trophoblastic neoplasms and increased thyroid activity. Typically, there were few, if any, symptoms or signs which could be unequivocally attributed to hyperthyroidism. All patients had tachycardia, but they were anemic, and most had pulmonary metastases. A widened pulse pressure and minor skin changes were present in about half of the cases. The basal metabolic rate, thyroidal uptake of ^{131}I, and serum thyroxine concentrations were usually elevated. Plasma TSH levels assessed by bioassay were high, but on radioimmunoassay they were undetectable.

Although M-TSH is distinct from the HCT formed in normal chorionic tissue, it is arguable whether the secretion of thyrotropin by trophoblastic tumors should be classified as ectopic production of a hormone. It is uncertain whether nontrophoblastic tumors ever produce ectopic TSH. A high concentration of TSH-like material was isolated from a poorly differentiated bronchial epidermoid epithelioma, but the patient was not clinically hyperthyroid.[185]

XI. CALCITONIN

Hall et al.[186] described three cases of breast cancer with symptomatic hypocalcemia, and postulated that the mechanism was the ectopic production of calcitonin by the tumor. However, the first case in which this was actually demonstrated was reported by Silva et al.[10] The patient had an oat-cell carcinoma of the bronchus, was normocalcemic, but had a high serum calcitonin level which fell after chemotherapy. The fact that the source of the hormone was ectopic was supported by the presence of a prominent arteriovenous gradient in calcitonin concentration across the tumor vascular bed.

Ectopic calcitonin production has now been observed in carcinoma of the bronchus,[20,187] breast cancer,[15,20] malignant melanoma,[188-190] pheochromocytoma,[188,190-191] islet cell tumors of the pancreas,[188,189] a mucosal neuroma,[191] and malignant melanoma.[188]

Calcitonin is normally produced by the parafollicular C cells of the thyroid gland; increased levels in medullary thyroid carcinoma do not, therefore, represent ectopic hormone production. However, the C cells do have the characteristics of the APUD series, and so, if the APUD hypothesis (Section I.C.2) is correct, ectopic calcitonin synthesis should occur in tumors derived from this cytological group. To a degree, this is true; typical examples are pheochromocytoma, malignant carcinoid, melanoma, and insulinoma. Abe et al.[190] examined tumors for their calcitonin content, and analyzed the results according to whether or not the tumors were derived from the APUD series. Included in the former group were medullary carcinomas of the thyroid, small-cell carcinomas of the lung, malignant carcinoids, pheochromocytomas, and a melanoma. Of these tumors, 97% contained immunoreactive calcitonin — 95% when the thyroid medullary carcinomas were excluded from the group. Of the nonAPUD group of tumors, only 37% contained calcitonin. The major inconsistency in relation to the APUD hypothesis is the high frequency of calcitonin-producing breast cancers and squamous bronchial carcinomas.

The ectopic origin of calcitonin in some cancers has been demonstrated by in vitro studies. Coombes et al.[15] observed secretion of the hormone by breast carcinoma cells in monolayer culture, and its production by breast cancer tissue passaged in "nude" mice. A cell line established in culture from a poorly differentiated epidermoid lung cancer produced both immunoreactive calcitonin and carcinoembryonic antigen.[16] The secreted calcitonin had a higher molecular weight than monomeric human calcitonin,[193] which is in keeping with some immunological differences between immunoreactive calcitonin in breast carcinoma tissue compared with synthetic human calcitonin.[194]

Calcitonin is not detectable by currently available assays in plasma or serum from normal adult subjects.[20] Coombes et al.[20] reported high plasma levels in 8 of 11 patients with oat-cell bronchial carcinomas, but none of four squamous-cell carcinomas of the bronchus. All of eight patients with breast cancer and bone involvement had detectable plasma calcitonin concentrations, and there was also a relationship between the presence of bone metastases and increased calcitonin production in the lung cancer patients. This may have been merely a reflection of the tumor cell mass required to produce sufficient of the hormone to elevate its circulating concentration to assayable levels.

In a later study,[15] 23 out of 28 patients with metastatic breast cancer (82%), but only 1 of 13 with disease restricted to the breast and regional lymph nodes had detectable levels of plasma calcitonin. It appears from these results that plasma calcitonin assays have a potential use in following tumor response to therapy, but not for the detection of very early disease. Hypercalcitoninemia is not usually associated with clinical manifestations.

XII. PROLACTIN AND PROLACTIN-RELEASING ACTIVITY

Ectopic production of prolactin has been reported in at least three cancer patients.

Turkington[14] described a woman with a renal-cell carcinoma, galactorrhea, and hyper-prolactinemia. Surgical resection of the tumor produced a prompt reduction in serum prolactin to normal levels, and ectopic secretion of the hormone was confirmed by the demonstration of its synthesis in tissue culture. When 21 lung cancer patients were screened for hyperprolactinemia, one, a male with an undifferentiated tumor, was found to have an elevated serum prolactin level. This was corrected after radiation therapy.[14]

The third case described by Rees et al.[17] has been referred to several times already in this review. The patient had an oat-cell carcinoma of the bronchus, in which was demonstrated ACTH, β-MSH, arginine vasopressin, corticotropin-like intermediate lobe peptide, and prolactin. Although ACTH and vasopressin production occurred in cell culture, there was no detectable prolactin secretion.

A single case has been reported of a medullary carcinoma of the thyroid with Cushing's syndrome and galactorrhea.[52] The tumor was ectopically producing not prolactin, but a prolactin production-stimulating factor, the activity of which was shown by the effect of tumor extracts on cultured rat pituitary cells.

XIII. GROWTH HORMONE AND GROWTH HORMONE-RELEASING HORMONE

The association of carcinoid tumors with acromegaly is well recognized, but, usually, it is part of a pleuriglandular syndrome in which the acromegaly is due to a mixed pituitary adenoma. Additional features may include primary hyperparathyroidism and hyperinsulinemia due to a pancreatic islet cell tumor.[195,196] Aside from these cases, acromegaly has been associated with the ectopic production of immunoreactive human growth hormone (IRHGH) or of growth hormone-releasing hormone by tumors.

Some patients with carcinoma of the bronchus have elevated plasma IRHGH levels, a failure of the normal suppression of IRHGH after glucose loading, and abnormal glucose tolerance;[197] frequently these hormonal changes are accompanied by hypertrophic pulmonary osteoarthropathy.[198-201] Although surgical removal of the tumor may be followed by improvement in the hypertrophic pulmonary osteoarthropathy, with a concomitant reduction in plasma IRHGH, there is considerable doubt that excessive growth-hormone activity is responsible for this clinical abnormality.[2,198,199] The significance of the failure of glucose to suppress IRHGH is unclear; paradoxical rises in the hormone after glucose loading also occur in cancer of the breast, and were attributed to a nonspecific stress response,[202] and in endometrial carcinoma.[203]

Ectopically produced IRHGH appears to be immunologically and chemically similar to human pituitary growth hormone. Greenberg et al.[201] studied a patient with an anaplastic large-cell carcinoma of the bronchus and hypertrophic pulmonary osteoarthropathy. The circulating concentration of IRHGH was elevated, and a tumor extract contained a high level of the polypeptide, compared with adjacent normal lung tissue. Tumor cells were established in long-term culture. They incorporated ^{14}C-leucine into HGH-like material; release of the hormone from tumor cells was stimulated by theophylline and 3'5' dibutyryl cyclic AMP, but not by a sheep growth hormone-releasing factor. In this respect, the tumor cells behaved in the same manner as pituitary growth hormone-secreting cells.

Davek[204] described two patients with bronchial carcinoids and acromegaly. Prior to surgery, both had elevated IRHGH levels in plasma, which were unsuppressible by glucose loading. After resection of the tumor, the plasma IRHGH concentrations were normal. Only one of the two tumors contained IRHGH, and it was postulated that in the other, ectopic synthesis of growth hormone-releasing factor may have been responsible for the endocrinopathy. The presence of growth hormone-releasing hormone has been demonstrated in lung cancer extracts,[205] and also in pulmonary carcinoid associated with acromegaly.[206]

REFERENCES

1. **Liddle, G. W., Island, D., and Meador, C. K.,** Normal and abnormal regulation of corticotropin secretion in man, *Recent Progr. Horm. Res.,* 18, 125, 1962.
2. **Rees, L. H.,** The biosynthesis of hormones by non-endocrine tumours — a review, *J. Endocrinol.,* 67, 143, 1975.
3. **Lewis, A. A. M. and Deshpande, N.,** The effect of hypophysectomy on the cortisol secretion in 4 patients with advanced metastatic breast cancer, *Br. J. Surg.,* 60, 493, 1973.
4. **Mason, A. M. S., Ratcliffe, J. G., Buckle, R. M., and Mason, A. S.,** ACTH secretion by bronchial carcinoid tumours, *Clin. Endocrinol.,* 1, 3, 1972.
5. **Scholz, D. A., Riggs, B. L., Purnell, D. C., Goldsmith, R. S., and Arnaud, C. D.,** Ectopic hyperparathyroidism with renal calculi and subperiosteal bone resorption, *Mayo Clin. Proc.,* 48, 124, 1973.
6. **Bower, B. F., Mason, D. M., and Forsham, P. H.,** Bronchogenic carcinoma with inappropriate antidiuretic activity in plasma and tumor, *N. Engl. J. Med.,* 271, 934, 1964.
7. **Faiman, C., Colwell, J. A., Ryan, R. J., Hershman, J. M., and Shields, T. W.,** Gonadotropin secretion from a bronchogenic carcinoma, *N. Engl. J. Med.,* 277, 1395, 1967.
8. **Ratcliffe, J. G., Scott, A. P., Bennett, H. P. J., Lowry, P. J., McMartin, C., Strong, J. A., and Walbaum, P. R.,** Production of corticotrophin-like intermediate lobe peptide and of corticotrophin by a bronchial carcinoid tumour, *Clin. Endocrinol.,* 2, 51, 1973.
9. **Buckle, R. M., McMillan, M., and Mallison, C.,** Ectopic secretion of parathyroid hormone by a renal adenocarcinoma in a patient with hypercalcemia, *Br. Med. J.,* 4, 724, 1970.
10. **Silva, O. L., Becker, K. L., Primack, A., Doppman, J., and Snider, R. H.,** Ectopic production of calcitonin, *Lancet,* 2, 317, 1973.
11. **Unger, R. H., Lochner, J. de V., and Eisentraut, A. M.,** Identification of insulin and glucagon in a bronchogenic metastasis, *J. Clin. Endocrinol. Metab.,* 24, 823, 1964.
12. **Holdaway, U. M. and Friesen, H. G.,** Hormone binding by human mammary carcinoma, *Cancer Res.,* 37, 1946, 1977.
13. **Tashjian, A. H., Jr.,** Animal cell cultures as a source of hormones, *Biotechnol. Bioeng.,* 11, 109, 1969.
14. **Turkington, R. W.,** Ectopic production of prolactin, *N. Engl. J. Med.,* 285, 1455, 1971.
15. **Coombes, R. C., Easty, G. C., Detre, S. I., Hillyard, C. J., Stevens, U., Girgis, S. I., Galante, L. S., Heywood, L., MacIntyre, I., and Neville, A. M.,** Secretion of immunoreactive calcitonin by human breast carcinomas, *Br. Med. J.,* 4, 197, 1975.
16. **Ellison, M., Woodhouse, D., Hillyard, C., Dowsett, M., Coombes, R. C., Gilby, E. D., Greenberg, P. B., and Neville, A. M.,** Immunoreactive calcitonin production by human lung carcinoma cells in culture, *Br. J. Cancer,* 32, 373, 1975.
17. **Rees, L. H., Bloomfield, G. A., Rees, G. M., Corrin, B., Franks, L. M., and Ratcliffe, J. G.,** Multiple hormones in a bronchial tumor, *J. Clin. Endocrinol. Metab.,* 38, 1090, 1974.
18. **Tormey, D. C. and Waalkes, T. P.,** Biochemical markers in cancer of the breast, in *Recent Results in Cancer Research,* 161, 57, Arneault, G. St., Band, P., and Israel, L., Eds., Springer-Verlag, Berlin, 1976, 78.
19. **Sheth, N. A., Suraiya, J. N., Sheth, A. R., Ranadive, K. J., and Jussawalla, D. J.,** Ectopic production of human placental lactogen by human breast tumors, *Cancer (Philadelphia),* 39, 1693, 1977.
20. **Coombes, R. C., Hillyard, C., Greenberg, P. B., and MacIntyre, I.,** Plasmaimmunoreactive-calcitonin in patients with non-thyroid tumors, *Lancet,* 1, 1080, 1974.
21. **Williams, E. D.,** Tumours, hormones and cellular differentiation, *Lancet,* 2, 1108, 1969.
22. **Pearse, A. G. E.,** The cytochemistry and ultrastructure of polypeptide hormone-producing cells of the APUD series and the embryologic, physiological and pathologic implications of the concept, *J. Histochem. Cytochem.,* 17, 303, 1969.
23. **Pearse, A. G. E. and Welbourn, R.,** The apudomas, *Br. J. Hosp. Med.,* 10, 617, 1973.
24. **Pearse, A. G. E. and Polak, J. M.,** Neural crest origin of the endocrine polypeptide (APUD) cells of the gastrointestinal tract and pancreas, *Gut,* 12, 783, 1971.

25. **Friesen, S. R., Hermreck, A. S., and Mantz, F. A.,** Glucagon, gastrin and carcinoid tumors of the duodenum, pancreas and stomach; polypeptide "apudomas" of the foregut, *Am. J. Surg.,* 127, 90, 1974.

26. **Pearse, A. G. E., Coulling, I., Weavers, B., and Friesen, S. R.,** The endocrine polypeptide cells of the human stomach, duodenum and jejunum, *Gut,* 11, 649, 1970.

27. **Bensch, K. G., Corrin, B., Pariente, R., and Spencer, H.,** Oat cell carcinoma of the lung. Its origin and relationship to bronchial carcinoid, *Cancer (Philadelphia),* 22, 1163, 1968.

28. **Baylin, S. B.,** Ectopic production of hormones and other proteins by tumors, *Hosp. Pract.,* 117, October 1975.

29. **Smith, L. H.,** Ectopic hormone production, *Surg. Gynecol. Obstet.,* 141, 443, 1975.

30. **Warner, T. F. C. S.,** Cell hybridization in the genesis of ectopic hormone-secreting tumours, *Lancet,* 1, 1259, 1974.

31. **Brown, W. H.,** A case of pleuriglandular syndrome — "Diabetes of bearded women," *Lancet,* 2, 1022, 1928.

32. **Liddle, G. W., Nicholson, W. E., Island, D. P., Orth, D. N., Abe, K., and Lowder, S. C.,** Clinical and laboratory studies of ectopic humoral syndromes, *Rec. Prog. Horm. Res.,* 25, 283, 1969.

33. **Kato, Y., Ferguson, T. B., Bennett, D. E., and Burford, T. H.,** Oat cell carcinoma of the lung. A review of 138 cases, *Cancer (Philadelphia),* 23, 517, 1969.

34. **Ross, E. J.,** Cancer and the adrenal cortex, *Proc. R. Soc. Med.,* 59, 335, 1966.

35. **Meador, C. K., Liddle, G. W., Island, D. P., Nicholson, W. E., Lucas, C. P., Nuckton, J. G., and Luetscher, J. A.,** Cause of Cushing's syndrome in patients with tumors arising from "nonendocrine" tissue, *J. Clin. Endocrinol. Metab.,* 22, 693, 1962.

36. **Liddle, G. W., Givens, J. R., Nicholson, W. E., and Island, D. P.,** The ectopic ACTH syndrome, *Cancer Res.,* 25, 1057, 1965.

37. **Orth, D. N., Nicholson, W. E., Mitchell, W. M., Island, D. P., and Liddle, G. W.,** Biologic and immunologic characterization and physical separation of ACTH and ACTH fragments in the ectopic ACTH syndrome, *J. Clin. Invest.,* 52, 1756, 1973.

38. **Ratcliffe, J. G., Knight, R. A., Besser, G. M., Landon, J., and Stansfeld, A. G.,** Tumour and plasma ACTH concentrations in patients with and without the ectopic ACTH syndrome, *Clin. Endocrinol.,* 1, 27, 1972.

39. **Orth, D. N.,** Establishment of human malignant melanoma clonal cell lines that secrete adrenocorticotrophin, *Nature (London), New Biol.,* 242, 26, 1973.

40. **Bloomfield, G. A., Holdaway, I. M., Corrin, B., Ratcliffe, J. G., Rees, G. M., Ellison, M., and Rees, L. H.,** Lung tumours and ACTH production, *Clin. Endocrinol.,* 6, 95, 1977.

41. **Scott, A. P., Bennett, H. P. J., Lowry, P. J., McMartin, C., and Ratcliffe, J. G.,** Corticotrophin-like intermediate-lobe peptide — a new pituitary and tumour peptide, *J. Endocrinol.,* 55, 36, 1972.

42. **Gewirtz, G., Schneider, B., Krieger, D. T., and Yalow, R. S.,** Big ACTH: conversion to biologically active ACTH by trypsin, *J. Clin. Endocrinol. Metab.,* 38, 227, 1974.

43. **Yalow, R. S. and Berson, S. A.,** Size heterogeneity of immunoreactive human ACTH in plasma and in extracts of pituitary glands and ACTH-producing thymoma, *Biochem. Biophys. Res. Commun.,* 44, 439, 1971.

44. **Yalow, R. S. and Berson, S. A.,** Characteristics of "big ACTH" in human plasma and pituitary extracts, *J. Clin. Endocrinol. Metab.,* 36, 415, 1973.

45. **Gewirtz, G. and Yalow, R. S.,** Ectopic ACTH production in carcinoma of the lung, *J. Clin. Invest.,* 53, 1022, 1974.

46. **McNamara, J. J., Varon, H. H., Paulson, D. L., Shah, I., and Urschel, H. C.,** Steroid hormone abnormalities in patients with carcinoma of the lung, *J. Thorac. Cardiovasc. Surg.,* 56, 371, 1968.

47. **Kawai, A., Tamura, M., Tanimoto, S., Honma, H., and Kuzuya, N.,** Studies on adrenal cortical function in patients with lung cancer, *Metabolism,* 18, 609, 1969.

48. **Imura, H., Matsukura, S., Yamamoto, H., Hirata, Y., Nakai, Y., Endo, J., Tanaka, A., and Nakamura, M.,** Studies on ectopic ACTH-producing tumors. II. Clinical and biochemical features of 30 cases, *Cancer (Philadelphia),* 35, 1430, 1975.

49. **Mason, A. S.,** Reflections on Cushing's syndrome, *Proc. R. Soc. Med.,* 64, 749, 1971.

50. **Friedman, M., Marshall-Jones, P., and Ross, E. J.,** Cushing's syndrome: adrenocortical hyperactivity secondary to neoplasms arising outside the pituitary-adrenal system, *Q. J. Med.,* 35, 193, 1966.

51. **Upton, G. V. and Amatruda, T. T., Jr.,** Evidence for the presence of tumor peptides with corticotropin-releasing factor-like activity in the ectopic ACTH syndrome, *N. Engl. J. Med.,* 285, 419, 1971.

52. **Birkenhäger, J. C., Upton, G. V., Seldenrath, H. J., Krieger, D. T., and Tashjian, A. H., Jr.,** Medullary thyroid carcinoma: ectopic production of peptides with ACTH-like, corticotrophin releasing factor-like and prolactin production-stimulating activities, *Acta Endocrinol. (Copenhagen),* 83, 280, 1976.

53. Landon, J., James, V. H. T., and Peart, W. S., Cushing's syndrome associated with a "corticotro-phin"-producing bronchial neoplasm, *Acta Endocrinol. (Copenhagen),* 56, 321, 1967.

54. Yamamoto, H., Hirata, Y., Matsukura, S., Imura, H., Nakamura, M., and Tanaka, A., Studies on ectopic ACTH-producing tumours. IV. CRF-like activity in tumour tissue, *Acta Endocrinol. (Copenhagen),* 82, 183, 1976.

55. Suda, T., Demura, H., Demura, R., Wakabayashi, I., Nomura, K., Odagiri, E., and Shizume, K., Corticotropin-releasing factor-like activity in ACTH producing tumors, *J. Clin. Endocrinol. Metab.,* 44, 440, 1977.

56. Sachs, B. A., Becker, N., Bloomberg, A. E., and Grunwald, R. P., "Cure" of ectopic ACTH syndrome secondary to adenocarcinoma of the lung, *J. Clin. Endocrinol. Metab.,* 30, 590, 1970.

57. Steel, K., Baerg, R. D., and Adams, D. O., Cushing's syndrome in association with a carcinoid tumor of the lung, *J. Clin. Endocrinol. Metab.,* 27, 1285, 1967.

58. Coll, R., Horner, I., Kraiem, Z., and Gafni, J., Successful metapyrone therapy of the ectopic ACTH syndrome, *Arch. Int. Med.,* 121, 549, 1968.

59. Carey, R. M., Orth, D. N., and Hartman, W. H., Malignant melanoma with ectopic production of ACTH: palliative treatment with inhibitors of adrenal steroid biosynthesis, *J. Clin. Endocrinol. Metab.,* 36, 482, 1973.

60. Hallwright, G. P., North, K. A. K., and Reid, J. D., Pigmentation and Cushing's syndrome due to a malignant tumor of the pancreas, *J. Clin. Endocrinol. Metab.,* 24, 496, 1964.

61. Island, D.P., Shimizu, N., Nicholson, W. E., Abe, K., Ogata, E. and Liddle, G. W., A method of separating small quantities of MSH and ACTH with good recovery of each, *J. Clin. Endocrinol. Metab.,* 25, 975, 1965.

62. Shimizu, N., Ogata, E., Nicholson, W. E., Island, D. P., Ney, R. L., and Liddle, G. W., Studies on the melanotrophic activity of human plasma and tissue, *J. Clin. Endocrinol. Metab.,* 25, 984, 1965.

63. Law, D. A., Liddle, G. W., Scott, H. W., and Tauber, S. D., Ectopic production of multiple hormones (ACTH, MSH and gastrin) by a single malignant tumor, *N. Engl. J. Med.,* 273, 292, 1965.

64. Hirata, Y., Matsukura, S., Imura, H., Yakura, T., Ihjima, S., Nagase, C., and Itoh, M., Two cases of multiple hormone-producing small cell carcinoma of the lung, *Cancer (Philadelphia),* 38, 2575, 1976.

65. Abe, K., Nicholson, W. E., Liddle, G. W., Island, D. P., and Orth, D. N., Radioimmunoassay for β-MSH in human plasma and tissues, *J. Clin. Invest.,* 46, 1609, 1967.

66. Gilkes, J. J. H., Bloomfield, G. A., Scott, A. P., Lowry, P. J., Ratcliffe, J. G., Landon, J., and Rees, L. H., Development and validation of a radioimmunoassay for peptides related to β-melanocyte stimulating hormone in human plasma; the lipotropins, *J. Clin. Endocrinol. Metab.,* 40, 450, 1975.

67. Bloomfield, G. A., Scott, A. P., Rees, L. H., Lowry, P. J., and Ratcliffe, J. G., ACTH and β-MSH related peptides in tumours associated with ectopic ACTH syndrome, *Acta Endocrinol. (Copenhagen), Suppl.,* 177, 148, 1973.

68. Bloomfield, G. A. and Scott, A. P., β-Melanocyte-stimulating hormone, *Proc. R. Soc. Med.,* 67, 748, 1974.

69. Bloomfield, G. A., Scott. A. P., Lowry, P. J., Gilkes, J. J. H., and Rees, L. H., A reappraisal of human βMSH, *Nature (London),* 252, 492, 1974.

70. Tanaka, K., Mount, C. D., Nicholson, W. E., and Orth, D. N., "Big" bioactive and immunoreactive "β-MSHs" in human plasma and tumor tissues, *Clin. Res.,* 24 (Abstr.), 10A, 1976.

71. Schwartz, W. B., Bennett, W., Curelop, S., and Bartter, F. C., A syndrome of renal sodium loss and hyponatremia probably resulting from inappropriate secretion of antidiuretic hormone, *Am. J. Med.,* 23, 529, 1957.

72. Amatruda, T. T., Jr., Mulrow, P. J., Gallagher, J. C., and Sawyer, W. H., Carcinoma of the lung with inappropriate antidiuresis, *N. Engl. J. Med.,* 269, 544, 1963.

73. Lebacq, E. and Delaere, J., Origine des substances antidiurétiques et explication de l'hypernatriurie dans le syndrome de Schwartz-Bartter, *Ann. Endocrinol. (Paris),* 26, 375, 1965.

74. Marks, L. J., Berde, B., Klein, L. A., Roth, J., Goonan, S. R., Blumen, D., and Nasbeth, D. C., Inappropriate vasopressin secretion and carcinoma of the pancreas, *Am. J. Med.,* 45, 967, 1968.

75. Vorherr, H., Massry, S. G., Utiger, R. D., and Kleeman, C. R., Antidiuretic principle in malignant tumor extracts from patients with inappropriate ADH syndrome, *J. Clin. Endocrinol. Metab.,* 28, 162, 1968.

76. Hamilton, B. P. M., Upton, G. V., and Amatruda, T. T., Jr., Evidence for the presence of neuro-physin in tumors producing the syndrome of inappropriate antidiuresis, *J. Clin. Endocrinol. Metab.,* 35, 764, 1972.

77. De Troyer, A. and Demanet, J. C., Clinical, biological and pathogenic features of the syndrome of inappropriate secretion of antidiuretic hormone, *Q. J. Med.,* 45, 521, 1976.

78. **Lipscombe, H. S., Wilson, C., Retiene, K., Matsen, F., and Ward, D. N.,** The syndrome of inappropriate secretion of antidiuretic hormone. A case report and characterization of an antidiuretic hormone-like material isolated from an oat cell carcinoma of the lung, *Cancer Res.*, 28, 378, 1968.

79. **Utiger, R. D.,** Inappropriate antidiuresis and carcinoma of the lung: detection of arginine vasopressin in tumor extracts by immunoassay, *J. Clin. Endocrinol. Metab.*, 26, 970, 1966.

80. **George, J. M., Capen, C. C., and Phillips, A. S.,** Biosynthesis of vasopressin in vitro and ultrastructure of a bronchogenic carcinoma, *J. Clin. Invest.*, 51, 141, 1972.

81. **Acher, R., Manoussos, G., and Olivry, G.,** Sur les relations entre l'octyocine et la vasopressine d'une part et la protéine de Van Dyke d'autre part, *Biochim. Biophys. Acta*, 16, 155, 1955.

82. **Barraclough, M. A., Jones, J. J., and Lee, J.,** Production of vasopressin by anaplastic oat cell carcinoma of the bronchus, *Clin. Sci.*, 31, 135, 1966.

83. **Beardwell, C. G.,** Radioimmunoassay of arginine vasopressin in human plasma, *J. Clin. Endocrinol. Metab.*, 33, 254, 1971.

84. **Rees, J. R., Rosalki, S. B., and MacLean, A. D. W.,** Hyponatraemia and impaired renal tubular function with carcinoma of bronchus, *Lancet*, 2, 1005, 1960.

85. **Daly, J. J., Nelson, M. A., and Rose, D. P.,** Hyponatraemia with carcinoma of the bronchus, *Postgrad. Med.*, 39, 158, 1963.

86. **Ross, E. J.,** Hyponatraemic syndromes associated with carcinoma of the bronchus, *Q. J. Med.*, 32, 297, 1963.

87. **Tisher, C. C.,** Correction of an ADH syndrome by resection of a bronchogenic carcinoma with demonstration of tumor antidiuretic activity, *Clin. Res.*, 14, 185, 1966.

88. **Bartter, F. C. and Schwartz, W. B.,** The syndrome of inappropriate secretion of antidiuretic hormone, *Am. J. Med.*, 42, 790, 1967.

89. **Hantmann, D. Rossier, B., Zohlman, R., and Schrier, R.,** Rapid correction of hyponatremia in the syndrome of inappropriate secretion of antidiuretic hormone, *Ann. Int. Med.*, 78, 870, 1973.

90. **Fusco, F. D. and Rosen, S. W.,** Gonadotropin-producing anaplastic large-cell carcinomas of lung, *N. Engl. J. Med.*, 275, 507, 1966.

91. **Becker, K. L., Cottrell, J., Moore, C. F., Winacker, J. L., Matthews, M. J., and Katz, S.,** Endocrine studies in a patient with a gonadotropin-secreting bronchogenic carcinoma, *J. Clin. Endocrinol. Metab.*, 28, 809, 1968.

92. **Dailey, J. E. and Marcuse, P. M.,** Gonadotropin secreting giant cell carcinoma of the lung, *Cancer (Philadelphia)*, 24, 388, 1969.

93. **Cottrell, J. C., Becker, K. L., Matthews, M. J., and Moore, C.,** The histology of gonadotropin-secreting bronchogenic carcinoma, *Am. J. Clin. Pathol.*, 52, 720, 1969.

94. **Reeves, R. L., Tesluk, H., and Harrison, C. E.,** Precocious puberty associated with hepatoma, *J. Clin. Endocrinol. Metab.*, 19, 1651, 1959.

95. **Behrle, F. C., Mantz, F. A., Olson, R. L., and Trombold, J. C.,** Virilization accompanying hepatoblastoma, *Pediatrics*, 32, 265, 1963.

96. **Root, A. W., Bongiovanni, A. M., and Eberlein, W. R.,** A testicular — interstitial-cell stimulating gonadotrophin in a child with hepatoblastoma and sexual precocity, *J. Clin. Endocrinol. Metab.*, 28, 1317, 1968.

97. **McArthur, J. W., Toll, G. D., Russfield, A. B., Reiss, A. M., Quinby, W. C., and Baker, W. H.,** Sexual precocity attributable to ectopic gonadotropin secretion by hepatoblastoma, *Am. J. Med.*, 54, 390, 1973.

98. **Omenn, G. S.,** Ectopic hormone syndromes associated with tumors in childhood, *Pediatrics*, 47, 613, 1971.

99. **Rosen, S. W. and Weintraub, B. D.,** Ectopic production of the isolated alpha subunit of the glycoprotein hormones, *N. Engl. J. Med.*, 290, 1441, 1974.

100. **Weintraub, B. D. and Rosen, S. W.,** Ectopic production of chorionic somatomammotropin by nontrophoblastic cancers, *J. Clin. Endocrinol. Metab.*, 32, 94, 1971.

101. **Rabson, A. S., Rosen, S. W., Tashjian, A. H., and Weintraub, B. D.,** Production of human chorionic gonadotrophin in vitro by a cell line derived from carcinoma of the lung, *J. Natl. Cancer Inst.*, 50, 669, 1973.

102. **Tashjian, A. H., Weintraub, B. D., Barowsky, N. J., Rabson, A.S., and Rosen, S. W.,** Subunits of human chorionic gonadotropin; unbalanced synthesis and secretion by clonal cell strains derived from a bronchogenic carcinoma, *Proc. Natl. Acad. Sci. U.S.A.*, 70, 1419, 1973.

103. **Anon.,** Case Records of the Massachusetts General Hospital (Case 39061), *N. Engl. J. Med.*, 225, 789, 1941.

104. **Conner, T. B., Thomas, W. C., Jr., and Howard, J. E.,** Etiology of hypercalcemia associated with lung carcinoma, *J. Clin. Invest.*, 35, 697, 1956.

105. **Plimpton, C. H. and Gellhorn, A.,** Hypercalcemia in malignant disease without evidence of bone destruction, *Am. J. Med.,* 21, 750, 1956.
106. **Omenn, G. S., Roth, S.I., and Baker, W. H.,** Hyperparathyroidism associated with malignant tumors of nonparathyroid origin, *Cancer (Philadelphia),* 24,1004, 1969.
107. **Rosen, S. W. and Weintraub, B. D.,** Ectopic gonadotropin in bronchogenic carcinoma, *JAMA,* 210, 908, 1969.
108. **Tashjian, A. H., Jr., Levine, L., and Munson, P. L.,** Immunochemical identification of parathyroid hormone in non-parathyroid neoplasms associated with hypercalcemia, *J. Exp. Med.,* 119, 467, 1964.
109. **Grimes, B. J., Fisher, B., Finn, F., and Danowski, T. S.,** Steroid-resistant hypercalcaemia and parathyroid hyperplasia in non-osseous cancer, *Acta Endocrinol.,* 56, 510, 1967.
110. **Sherwood, L. M., O'Riordan, J. L. H., Aurbach, G. D. and Potts, J. T., Jr.,** Production of parathyroid hormone by non-parathyroid tumors, *J. Clin. Endocrinol. Metab.,* 27, 140, 1967.
111. **Knill-Jones, R. P., Buckle, R. M., Parsons, V., Calne, R. Y., and Williams, R.,** Hypercalemia and increased parathyroid-hormone activity in a primary hepatoma. Studies before and after hepatic transplantation, *N. Engl. J. Med.,* 282, 704, 1970.
112. **Mavligit, G. M., Cohen, J. L., and Sherwood, L. M.,** Ectopic production of parathyroid hormone by carcinoma of the breast, *N. Engl. J. Med.,* 285, 154, 1971.
113. **Melick, R. A., Martin, T. J., and Hicks, J. D.,** Parathyroid hormone production and malignancy, *Br. Med. J.,* 2, 204, 1972.
114. **Munson, P. L., Tashjian, A. H., and Levine, L.,** Evidence for parathyroid hormone in nonparathyroid tumors associated with hypercalcemia, *Cancer Res.,* 25, 1062, 1965.
115. **Riggs, B. L., Arnaud, D. C., Reynolds, J. C., and Smith, L. H.,** Immunologic differentiation of primary hyperparathyroidism from hyperparathyroidism due to nonparathyroid cancer, *J. Clin. Invest.,* 50, 2079, 1971.
116. **Benson, R. C., Jr., Riggs, L., Pickard, B. M., and Arnaud, C. D.,** Immunoreactive forms of circulating parathyroid hormone in primary and ectopic hyperparathyroidism, *J. Clin. Invest.,* 54, 175, 1974.
117. **Kemper, B., Habener, J. F., Mulligan, R. C., Potts, J. T., and Rich, A.,** Pre-proparathyroid hormone — a direct translation product of parathyroid messenger RNA, *Proc. Natl. Acad. Sci. U.S.A.,* 71, 3731, 1974.
118. **Lafferty, F. W.,** Pseudohyperparathyroidism, *Medicine,* 45, 247, 1966.
119. **Liddle, G. W. and Ball, J. H.,** Manifestations of cancer mediated by ectopic hormones, in *Cancer Medicine,* Holland, J. F. and Frei, E., Eds., Lea & Febiger, Philadelphia, 1973, 1046.
120. **Klein, D. C. and Raisz, L. G.,** Prostaglandins: stimulation of bone resorption in tissue culture, *Endocrinology,* 86, 1436, 1970.
121. **Tashjian, A. H., Jr., Voelkel, E. F., Levine, L., and Goldhaber, P.,** Evidence that the bone resorption-stimulating factor produced by mouse fibrosarcoma cells is prostaglandin E_2: a new model for the hypercalcemia of cancer, *J. Exp. Med.,* 136, 1329, 1972.
122. **Tashjian, A. H., Jr., Voelkel, E. F., Goldhaber, P., and Levine, L.,** Prostaglandins, calcium metabolism and cancer, *Fed. Proc.,* 33, 81, 1974.
123. **Voelkel, E. F., Tashjian, A. H., Jr., Franklin, R., Wasserman, E., and Levine, L.,** Hypercalcemia and tumor-prostaglandins: the VX_2 carcinoma model in the rabbit, *Metabolism,* 24, 973, 1975.
124. **Powell, D., Singer, F. R., Murray, T. M., Minkin, C., and Potts, J. T. Jr.,** Nonparathyroid humoral hypercalcemia in patients with neoplastic diseases, *N. Engl. J. Med.,* 289, 176, 1973.
125. **Powles, T. J., Clark, S. A., Easty, D. M., Easty, G. C., Munro, N., Neville, A.,** The inhibition by aspirin and indomethacin of osteolytic tumour deposits and hypercalcaemia in rats with Walker tumour, and its possible application to human breast cancer, *Br. J. Cancer,* 28, 316, 1973.
126. **Galasko, C. S. B. and Bennett, A.,** Relationship of bone destruction in skeletal metastases to osteoclast activation and prostaglandins, *Nature (London),* 263, 508, 1976.
127. **Brereton, H. D., Halushka, P. V., Alexander, R. W., Mason, D. M., Keiser, H. R., and DeVita, V. T.,** Indomethacin-responsive hypercalcemia in a patient with renal-cell adenocarcinoma, *N. Engl. J. Med.,* 291, 83, 1974.
128. **Robertson, R. P., Baylink, D. J., Marini, J.J., and Adkison, H. W.,** Elevated prostaglandins and suppressed parathyroid hormone associated with hypercalcemia and renal cell carcinoma, *J. Clin. Endocrinol. Metab.,* 41, 164, 1975.
129. **Robertson, R. P., Baylink, D. J., Metz, S. A., and Cummings, K. B.,** Plasma prostaglandin E in patients with cancer with and without hypercalcemia, *J. Clin. Endocrinol. Metab.,* 43, 1330, 1976.
130. **Cummings, K. B., Wheelis, R. F., and Robertson, R. P.,** Prostaglandin: increased production by renal cell carcinoma, *Surg. Forum,* 26, 572, 1975.
131. **Seyberth, H. W., Segre, G. V., Morgan, J. L., Sweetman, B. J., Potts, J. T., and Oates, J. A.,** Prostaglandins as mediators of hypercalcemia associated with certain types of cancer, *N. Engl. J. Med.,* 293, 1278, 1975.

132. Powles, T. J., Dowsett, M., Easty, D. M., Easty, G. C., Neville, A. M., Breast cancer osteolysis, bone metastases, and anti-osteolytic effect of aspirin, *Lancet*, 1, 608, 1976.

133. Bennett, A., McDonald, A. M., Simpson, J. S., and Stamford, I. F., Breast cancer, prostaglandins, and bone metastases, *Lancet*, 1, 1218, 1975.

134. Bennett, A., Charlier, E. M., McDonald, A. M., Simpson, J. S., Stamford, I. F., and Zebro, T., Prostaglandins and breast cancer, *Lancet*, 2, 624, 1977.

135. Lipsett, M. B., Odell, W. D., Rosenberg, L. E., and Waldmann, T. A., Humoral syndromes associated with nonendocrine tumors, *Ann. Int. Med.*, 61, 733, 1964.

136. Floyd, J. C. Jr., Power, L., Rull, J., Fajans, S. S., and Conn, J. W., Insulin and ILA in tissue extracts and plasma of patients with nonpancreatic tumors associated with hypoglycemia, *Clin. Res.*, 11, 297, 1963.

137. Carey, R. W., Pretlow, T. G., Ezdinli, E. Z., and Holland, J. F., Studies on the mechanism of hypoglycemia in a patient with massive intraperitoneal leiomyosarcoma, *Am. J. Med.*, 40, 458, 1966.

138. Paullada, J. J., Lisci-Garmilla, A., Gonzáles-Angulo, A., Jurado-Mendoza, J., Quijano-Narezo, M., Gómez-Peralta, L., and Doria-Medina, M., Hemangiopericytoma associated with hypoglycemia, *Am. J. Med.*, 44, 990, 1968.

139. Shames, J. M., Dhurandhar, N. R., and Blackard, W. G., Insulin-secreting bronchial carcinoid tumor with widespread metastases, *Am. J. Med.*, 44, 632, 1968.

140. Kiang, D. T., Bauer, G. E., and Kennedy, B. J., Immunoassayable insulin in carcinoma of the cervix associated with hypoglycemia, *Cancer (Philadelphia)*, 31, 801, 1973.

141. Megyesi, K., Kahn, C. R., Roth, J., and Gorden, P., Hypoglycemia in association with extrapancreatic tumors: demonstration of elevated plasma NSILA-s by a new radioreceptor assay, *J. Clin. Endocrinol. Metab.*, 38, 931, 1974.

142. McFadzean, A. J. S. and Yeung, T. T., Hypoglycemia in primary carcinoma of the liver, *Arch. Int. Med.*, 98, 720, 1956.

143. Miller, D. W., Stewart, C. F., and Rosner, W., Hypoglycemia caused by abdominal leiomyosarcoma, *Am. J. Surg.*, 119, 754, 1970.

144. August, J. T. and Hiatt, H. H., Severe hypoglycemia secondary to a nonpancreatic fibrosarcoma with insulin activity, *N. Engl. J. Med.*, 258, 17, 1958.

145. Butterfield, W.J. H., Kinder, C. H., and Mahler, R. F., Hypoglycaemia associated with sarcoma, *Lancet*, 1, 703, 1960.

146. Silverstein, M. N., Wakim, K. G., Bahn, R. C., and Bayrd, E. D., A hypoglycemic factor in leukemic tumors, *Proc. Soc. Exp. Biol. Med.*, 103, 824, 1960.

147. Malpas, J. S., Blandford, G., White, R. J., and Wrigley, P. F. M., Some remote effects of "nonendocrine" cancer, *Proc. R. Soc. Med.*, 61, 463, 1968.

148. Hertko, E. J., Polycythemia (erythrocytosis) associated with uterine fibroids: a case report with erythropoietic activity demonstrated in the tumor, *Ann. Int. Med.*, 68, 1169, 1968.

149. Wrigley, P. F. M., Malpas, J. S., Turnbull, A. L., Jenkins, G. C., and McArt, A., Secondary polycythaemia due to a uterine fibromyoma producing erythropoietin, *Br. J. Haematol.*, 21, 551, 1971.

150. Ossias, A. L., Zanjani, E. D., Zalusky, R., Estren, S., and Wasserman, L. R., Case report: studies on the mechanism of erythrocytosis associated with a uterine fibromyoma, *Br. J. Haematol.*, 25, 179, 1973.

151. Waldmann, T. A., Rosse, W. F., and Swarm, R. L., The erythropoiesis-stimulating factors produced by tumors, *Ann. N. Y. Acad. Sci.*, 149, 509, 1968.

152. Schonfeld, A., Babbott, D., and Gundersen, K., Hypoglycemia and polycythemia associated with primary hepatoma, *N. Engl. J. Med.*, 265, 231, 1961.

153. Waldmann, T. A. and Bradley, J. E., Polycythemia secondary to a pheochromocytoma with production of an erythropoiesis stimulating factor by the tumor, *Proc. Soc. Exp. Biol. Med.*, 108, 425, 1961.

154. Shalet, M. F., Holder, T. M., and Walters, T. R., Erythropoietin-producing Wilms' tumor, *J. Pediatr.*, 70, 615, 1967.

155. Kenny, G. M., Mirand, E. A., Staubitz, W. J., Allen, J. E., Trudel, P. J., and Murphy, G. P., Erythropoietin levels in Wilms' tumor patients, *J. Urol.*, 104, 758, 1970.

156. Murphy, G. P., Mirand, E. A., and Staubitz, W. J., The value of erythropoietin assay in the follow-up of Wilms' tumor patients, *Oncology*, 33, 154, 1976.

157. Zollinger, R. M. and Ellison, E. H., Primary peptic ulceration of the jejunum associated with islet cell tumors of the pancreas, *Ann. Surg.*, 142, 709, 1955.

158. Hoffmann, J. W., Fox, P. S., and Wilson, S. D., Duodenal wall tumors and the Zollinger-Ellison syndrome; surgical management, *Arch. Surg.*, 107, 334, 1973.

159. Moshal, M. G., Broitman, S. A., and Zamcheck, N., Inhibition of glucose, water and electrolyte absorption by gastrin like pentapeptide (GLP), *Clin. Res.*, 17, 308, 1969.

160. **Yalow, R. S. and Berson, S. A.**, Size and charge distinctions between endogenous human plasma gastrin in peripheral blood and heptadecapeptide gastrins, *Gastroenterology*, 58, 609, 1970.
161. **Yalow, R. S. and Wu, N.**, Additional studies on the nature of big big gastrin, *Gastroenterology*, 65, 19, 1973.
162. **Gregory, R. A. and Tracy, H. J.**, The constitution and properties of two gastrins extracted from hog antral mucosa, *Gut*, 5, 103, 1964.
163. **Gregory, R. A., Tracy, H. J., Agarwal, K. L., and Grossman, M. I.**, Amino acid constitution of two gastrins isolated from Zollinger-Ellison tumour tissue, *Gut*, 10, 603, 1969.
164. **Yalow, R. S. and Berson, S. A.**, Nature of immunoreactive gastrin extracted from tissues of gastrointestinal tract, *Gastroenterology*, 60, 215, 1971.
165. **Gregory, R. A., and Tracy, H. J.**, The isolation of two "big gastrins" from Zollinger-Ellison tumour tissue, *Lancet*, 2, 797, 1972.
166. **Rehfeld, J. F. and Stadil, F.**, Gel filtration studies on immunoreactive gastrin in serum from Zollinger-Ellison patients, *Gut*, 14, 369, 1973.
167. **Said, S. I. and Mutt, V.**, Isolation from porcine-intestinal wall of a vasoactive octacosapeptide related to secretin and to glucagon, *Eur. J. Biochem.*, 28, 199, 1972.
168. **Bodansky, M., Klausner, Y. S., and Said, S. I.**, Biological activities of synthetic peptides corresponding to fragments of and to the entire sequence of the vasoactive intestinal peptide, *Proc. Natl. Acad. Sci.*, 70, 382, 1973.
169. **Bloom, S. R., Polak, J. M., and Pearse, A. G. E.**, Vasoactive intestinal peptide and watery-diarrhoea syndrome, *Lancet*, 2, 14, 1973.
170. **Said, S. I. and Faloona, G. R.**, Vasoactive intestinal peptide and watery diarrhea, *N. Engl. J. Med.*, 293, 155, 1975.
171. **Brown, J. C. and Dryburgh, J. R.**, A gastric inhibitory polypeptide II: the complete amino acid sequence, *Can. J. Biochem.*, 49, 865, 1971.
172. **Elias, E., Polak, J. M., Bloom, S. R., Pearse, A. G. E., Welbourne, R. B., Booth, C. C., Kuzio, M., and Brown, J. C.**, Pancreatic cholera due to production of gastric inhibitory polypeptide, *Lancet*, 2, 791, 1972.
173. **Gleeson, M. H., Bloom, S. R., Polak, J. M., Henry, K., and Dowling, R. H.**, Endocrine tumour in kidney affecting small bowel structure, motility, and absorptive function, *Gut*, 12, 773, 1971.
174. **Bloom, S. R.**, An enteroglucagon tumour, *Gut*, 13, 520, 1972.
175. **Hershman, J. M., Higgins, H. P., and Starnes, W. R.**, Differences between thyroid stimulator in hydatidiform mole and human chorionic thyrotropin, *Metabolism*, 19, 735, 1970.
176. **Hennen, G.**, Detection and study of a human-chorionic-thyroid-stimulating factor, *Arch. Int. Physiol. Biochim.*, 73, 689, 1965.
177. **Hennen, G., Pierce, J. G., and Freychet, P.**, Human chorionic thyrotropin further characterization and study of its secretion during pregnancy, *J. Clin. Endocrinol. Metab.*, 29, 581, 1969.
178. **Hershman, J. M. and Higgins, H. P.**, Hydatidiform mole — a cause of clinical hyperthyroidism, *N. Engl. J. Med.*, 284, 573, 1971.
179. **Dowling, J. T., Ingbar, S. H., and Freinkel, N.**, Iodine metabolism in hydatidiform mole and choriocarcinoma, *J. Clin. Endocrinol. Metab.*, 20, 1, 1960.
180. **Kock, H., Kessel, H. V., Stolte, L., and Levsden, H. V.**, Thyroid function in molar pregnancy, *J. Clin. Endocrinol. Metab.*, 26, 1128, 1966.
181. **Odell, W. D., Bates, R. W., Rivlin, R. S., Lipsett, M. B., and Hertz, R.**, Increased thyroid function without clinical hyperthyroidism in patients with choriocarcinoma, *J. Clin. Endocrinol. Metab.*, 23, 658, 1963.
182. **Odell, W. D., Hertz, R., Lipsett, M. B., Ross, G. T., and Hammond, C. B.**, Endocrine aspects of trophoblastic neoplasms, *Clin. Obstet. Gynecol.*, 10, 290, 1967.
183. **Steigbigel, N. H., Oppenheim, J. J., Fishman, L. M., and Carbone, P. P.**, Metastatic embryonal carcinoma of the testis associated with elevated plasma TSH-like activity and hyperthyroidism, *N. Engl. J. Med.*, 271, 345, 1964.
184. **Winand, R., Bates, R., Becker, C. E., and Rosen, S. W.**, Unusual thyroid-stimulating activity in the plasma of a man with choriocarcinoma, *J. Clin. Endocrinol. Metab.*, 29, 1369, 1969.
185. **Hennen, G.**, Characterization of a thyroid-stimulating factor in a human cancer tissue, *J. Clin. Endocrinol. Metab.*, 27, 610, 1967.
186. **Hall, T. C., Griffiths, C. T., and Petranek, J. R.**, Hypocalcemia — an unusual metabolic complication of breast cancer, *N. Engl. J. Med.*, 275, 1474, 1966.
187. **Whitelaw, A. G. L. and Cohen, S. L.**, Ectopic production of calcitonin, *Lancet*, 2, 443, 1973.
188. **Milhaud, G., Calmette, C., Taboulet, J., Julienne, A., and Moukhtar, M. S.**, Hypersecretion of calcitonin in neoplastic conditions, *Lancet*, 1, 462, 1974.
189. **Deftos, L. J., McMillan, P. J., Sartiano, G. P., Abuid, J., and Robinson, A. G.**, Simultaneous ectopic production of parathyroid hormone and calcitonin, *Metabolism*, 25, 543, 1976.

190. Abe, K., Adachi, I., Miyakawa, S., Tanaka, M., Yamaguchi, K., Tanaka, N., Kameya, T., and Shimosato, Y., Production of calcitonin, adrenocorticotropic hormone, and β- melanocyte-stimulating hormone in tumors derived from amine precursor uptake and decarboxylation cells, *Cancer Res.*, 37, 4190, 1977.

191. Voelkel, E. F., Tashjian, A. H., Jr., Davidoff, F. F., Cohen, R. B., Perlia, C. P., and Wurtman, R. J., Concentrations of calcitonin and catecholamines in phaeochromocytomas, a mucosal neuroma and medullary thyroid carcinoma, *J. Clin. Endocrinol. Metab.*, 37, 297, 1973.

192. Kalager, T., Glück, E., Heinmann, P., and Myking, O., Phaeochromocytoma with ectopic calcitonin production and parathyroid cyst, *Br. Med. J.*, 23, 21, 1977.

193. Coombes, R. C., Ellison, M. L., Girgis, S., Hillyard, C. J., MacIntyre, I., and Neville, A. M., The heterogeneity of human calcitonin secreted by human tumours, *In vitro*, in press.

194. Hillyard, C. J., Coombes, R. C., Greenberg, P. B., Galante, L. S., and MacIntyre, I., Calcitonin in breast and lung cancer, *Clin. Endocrinol.*, 5, 1, 1976.

195. Payne, W. S., Fontana, R. S., and Woolner, L. B., Bronchial tumors originating from mucous glands: current classification and unusual manifestations, *Med. Clin. North Am.*, 48, 945, 1964.

196. Williams, E. D. and Celestin, L. R., The association of bronchial carcinoid and pluriglandular adenomatosis, *Thorax*, 17, 120, 1962.

197. Sparagana, M., Phillips, G., Hoffman, C., and Kucera, L., Ectopic growth hormone syndrome associated with lung cancer, *Metabolism*, 20, 730, 1971.

198. Steiner, H., Dahlback, O., and Waldenstrom, J., Ectopic growth-hormone production and osteoarthropathy in carcinoma of the bronchus, *Lancet*, 1, 783, 1968.

199. Cameron, D. P., Burger, H. G., de Kretzer, D. M., Catt, K. J., and Best, J. B., On the presence of immunoreactive growth hormone in a bronchogenic carcinoma, *Australas. Ann. Med.*, 18, 143, 1969.

200. Dupont, B., Höyer, I., Borgeskov, S., and Nerup, S., Plasma growth hormone and hypertrophic osteoarthopathy in carcinoma of the bronchus, *Acta Med. Scand.*, 188, 25, 1970.

201. Greenberg, P. B., Beck, C., Martin, T. J., and Burger, H. G., Synthesis and release of human growth hormone from lung carcinoma in cell culture, *Lancet*, 1, 350, 1972.

202. Greenwood, F. C., James, V. H. T., Meggitt, B. F., Miller, J. D., and Taylor, P. H., Pituitary function in breast cancer, in *Prognostic Factors in Breast Cancer*, Forrest, A. P. M., and Kunkler, P. B., Eds., Livingstone, Edinburgh, 1968, 409.

203. Benjamin, F., Casper, D. J., Sherman, L., and Kolodny, H. D., Growth-hormone secretion in patients with endometrial carcinoma, *N. Engl. J. Med.*, 281, 1448, 1969.

204. Davek, J. T., Bronchial carcinoid with acromegaly in two patients, *J. Clin. Endocrinol. Metab.*, 38, 329, 1974.

205. Beck, C., Larkins, R. G., Martin, T. J., and Burger, H. G., Stimulation of growth hormone release from superfused rat pituitary by extracts of hypothalamus and of human lung tumours, *J. Endocrinol.*, 59, 325, 1973.

206. Sönksen, P. H., Ayres, A. B., Brainbridge, M., Corrin, B., Davies, D. R., Jeremiah, G. M., Oaten, S. W., Lowy, C., and West, T. E. T., Acromegaly caused by pulmonary carcinoid tumours, *Clin. Endocrinol.*, 5, 503, 1976.

Chapter 6

CIRCULATING TUMOR MARKERS

D. C. Tormey, A. S. Coates, and R. P. Whitehead

TABLE OF CONTENTS

I. INTRODUCTION

A circulating tumor marker can be defined as a substance present in a body fluid which qualitatively or quantitatively reflects the presence of malignancy. With currently available tumor markers, a compromise must be reached between sensitivity and specificity. Thus, if a threshold value is set low, elevated marker levels will be detected in a large percentage of patients with tumors, but this will be at the cost of an increased prevalence of elevated levels among patients without tumors. Conversely, if the threshold value is set high, the false positive rate will be reduced, but at the cost of reducing the prevalence of the elevated levels in patients where tumor is indeed present.

These considerations have limited the application of tumor markers in the screening process for tumor detection. Nevertheless, functionally useful compromise levels have been established which allow many of the markers a valuable role in the sequential assessment of tumor response and/or progression to therapy.

Although each marker has traditionally been considered for its value as a unique cancer indicator, it is clear that none presently meet that criterion (vide supra). Accordingly, attention has begun to be directed at using a matrix of tests with the hope of increasing both the sensitivity and specificity of their usefulness.

A great number of substances have been proposed as tumor markers. Many of these are either poorly characterized as markers, controversial, or have not been sufficiently examined. Such substances would include metabolic cations like zinc or copper, enzymes like serum glutamyl glycotransferase or serum lactate dehydrogenase, proteins not fully characterized, or nonspecific tests such as the erythrocyte sedimentation rate. Such markers will not be discussed in this chapter. As with any review, we regret the necessary arbitrariness and oversights that result in exclusions. With this recognition, it is our intent to review the origin, composition, and clinical usefulness of the currently available circulating tumor markers of major clinical utility.

II. ALPHA FETO-PROTEIN

Alpha Feto-Protein (AFP) is one of a group of oncofetal substances useful as tumor markers. Human embryonic cells present a full genetic complement of the information required for a variety of differentiated functions, but during differentiation, selected sections of the genome undergo a repressive process so that certain cellular components expressed during fetal development are either absent or present in very low amounts in the adult cells. During carcinogenesis, increased amounts of such substances may again be produced and function as tumor markers.

In 1963, Abelev et al.[1] developed antisera against the serum proteins of newborn mice and absorbed them with normal adult mouse serum. The absorbed antisera retained reactivity with newborn mouse serum, serum of adult mice bearing transplantable hepatomas, and normal adult mice that had undergone partial hepatectomies. A similar component has subsequently been detected in fetal blood and in the blood of hepatoma-bearing individuals of many other mammalian species, including man.[2] Human alpha feto-protein has a molecular weight of 64,000,[3] contains 4% carbohydrate, and has the electrophoretic mobility of an α_1 globulin.

Several assays are available for detection of AFP in human serum (Table 1). Although they vary considerably in their threshold of detection, the most sensitive technique is radioimmunoassay, which detects small amounts of AFP in the serum of normal adults. AFP is the major component during early fetal development and is detectable in human fetal serum from approximately the sixth week of gestation, reaching a peak at the 13th week. Thereafter, levels decline as albumin replaces AFP. Elevated levels of AFP are found in the serum of pregnant women, reaching 500 ng/mℓ during the third trimester. Higher levels have been used as an index of fetal distress or the presence of malformations such as a neural tube defect.[5-7]

The radioimmunoassay is the only method capable of detecting normal adult levels, which are usually less than 20 ng/mℓ. Waldmann and McIntire[8] used 40 ng/mℓ as the upper limit of normal and tested patients with various conditions for elevated values (Tables 2 and 3). Besides malignancy, elevated AFP levels were observed in pregnancy,

TABLE 1

Methods of Detection of Circulating AFP

Technique	Approximate threshold
Immunodiffusion in agar gel	1000—3000 ng/mℓ
Radioimmunodiffusion	100 ng/mℓ
Counterimmunoelectrophoresis	100 ng/mℓ
Passive hemagglutination	30 ng/mℓ
Radioimmunoassay	0.25 ng/mℓ

From Pick, A. I., Shoenfeld, Y., Schreibman, S., Weiss, H., and Ben-Bassat, M., *N.Y. State J. Med.*, 75, 1103, 1975. With permission.

TABLE 2

AFP Elevations in Nonmalignant Conditions

Diagnosis	Number of samples assayed	Percent of AFP values > 40 ng/mℓ
Normal adults	190	0
Normal children	20	0
Benign breast disease	112	0
Ulcerative colitis	30	0
Gastric ulcer	12	0
Duodenal ulcer	31	0
Chronic lung disease	16	0
Pneumonitis	10	0
Benign testicular disease	28	0
Immunodeficiency other than ataxia telangiectasia	42	0
Regional enteritis	19	(1)∿5
Pregnancy	—	(+)
Infants less than 1 year old	—	(+)
Classical viral hepatitis	—	27
Postnecrotic cirrhosis	—	24
Primary biliary cirrhosis	—	5
Active Laennec's cirrhosis	—	15
Ataxia telangiectasia	40	100

From Waldmann, T. A. and McIntire, K. R., *Cancer, Philadelphia,* 34, 1510, 1974. With permission.

infants under 1 year of age, some benign liver diseases associated with liver cell damage, and ataxia telangiectasia, an autosomal recessive immunodeficiency disorder that may be due to a defect in differentiation.

Other authors,[9] using 20 ng/mℓ as the upper limit of normal, found elevated AFP values in 1 of 26 cases of hemochromatosis, none of 50 cases of HB$_s$Ag antigen positive patients, and none of 26 patients with hematologic malignancies.

Waldmann and McIntire[8] reported a high percentage of patients with hepatocellular or testicular carcinoma with abnormal values when tested by radioimmunoassay (Table 3). Elevated AFP values were also found in patients with GI malignancies with or without evident hepatic metastases; thus, elevated levels do not always imply liver in-

TABLE 3

AFP Elevations in Malignant Conditions

Diagnosis	Number of Pts.	Percent of serum AFP values > 40 ng/ml
Hepatocellular carcinoma	130	72
Testicular teratocarcinoma and embryonal cell carcinoma	101	75
Pancreatic carcinoma	44	23
Gastric carcinoma	91	18
Colonic carcinoma	193	5
Bronchogenic carcinoma	150	7
Breast carcinoma	55	0
Nonhepatic benign lesions	300	0.3
Normal controls over 1 year of age	210	0
Biliary tract carcinoma[19]	8	25

From Waldmann, T. A. and McIntire, K. R., *Cancer (Philadelphia)*, 34, 1510, 1974. With permission.

volvement.[8] Malignant teratomas of ovary and mediastinum, as well as the testis, may be associated with elevated AFP levels,[9] but benign teratomas in patients over 1 year of age are usually associated with normal levels.[10] Any endodermal sinus tumor, including those arising in extra gonadal sites, may produce AFP.[11] High urinary AFP levels have been associated with high blood levels in nine patients with hepatoma.[12]

In an attempt to determine the usefulness of AFP in differentiating liver cirrhosis from hepatoma, Tonami et al.[13] compared AFP levels with liver scans. Using 200 ng/ml as the lower limit of AFP value in malignant liver disease, 21 of 27 cases of primary hepatocellular carcinoma were associated with high AFP levels. Only 5 of 153 cases of hepatitis and cirrhosis and 5 of 42 cases of stomach cancer had high values. The liver scan was abnormal in 22 of the 27 cases of primary liver carcinoma. In four cases with a positive scan, AFP was negative and in three cases with elevated AFP, the scan was negative. It appears that AFP may be elevated when there are lesions in the liver too small to show on scan; as such, these may be surgically curable when demonstrated by arteriography. AFP values may be as high as 1000 ng/ml in cirrhosis when no tumor can be found on scan, arteriogram, or clinical evaluation.[14]

While there is no overall correlation between AFP levels and the size of tumors in different patients, serial AFP levels in a given patient do appear to reflect the relative tumor burden of that patient's tumor, though in some patients AFP levels fall as a preterminal event.[15] Tumor removal by partial hepatectomy results in a rapid fall of serum AFP levels, while a later rise in the levels may precede clinically detectable tumor recurrence by 1 to 6 months.[15]

AFP levels can also be used to monitor therapy in patients with testicular choriocarcinoma, teratocarcinoma, and embryonal cell carcinoma, but not seminoma. Waldmann and McIntire[8] studied 14 such patients with disseminated tumors and elevated AFP. There was a reduction in AFP levels following clinically successful chemotherapy. AFP levels remaining elevated, even in the absence of clinical evidence of disease, presaged recurrence of tumor within the following 2 to 12 months.

In a study of 26 patients with embryonal cell carcinoma of the testis, Bourgeaux et al.[16] made many of the same observations. They found that high AFP levels were usually associated with or followed by multiple metastases and initially elevated AFP values indicated a poor prognosis. In many cases, serial AFP measurements reflected the response to chemotherapy and the clinical evolution of the disease.

III. CARCINO-EMBRYONIC ANTIGEN (CEA)

Carcino-embryonic antigen is another oncofetal antigen, first described in 1965 by Gold and Freedman.[17] They produced antisera to a saline extract of colonic carcinoma, which after appropriate absorptions, did not react with normal tissue, but produced a single precipitin line with tumor extracts. Identical reactivity was found in primary tumors of all levels of the GI tract from esophagus to rectum, including pancreas, and also in metastatic tumors from these primary sites. The substance was also found to be present in the fetal alimentary tract.

CEA is prepared by perchloric acid extraction of tumors, followed by sequential chromatographic purification. Although there is no international standard criterion of purity, the physical and chemical properties of CEA have recently been reviewed.[18] It is a glycoprotein of approximately 200,000 mol wt showing heterogeneity on isoelectric focusing due to variations in the amounts of carbohydrate present.[19] Cross reactivity with blood group A substance is present on some, but not all, preparations of CEA, and it has been shown that the antigenic site responsible for this cross reactivity is distinct from the specific CEA determinant.[18]

Studies using immunochemical microscopy approaches have demonstrated the presence of CEA at the cell surface and in the glycocalyx.[20,21] Small amounts of CEA are normally present in the lumen of the gastrointestinal tract and can be detected in feces. CEA is rapidly cleared from the circulation following injection into animals, with the major accumulation appearing in the liver.[22]

A variety of radioimmunoassay methods have been used for the detection and measurement of CEA in the circulation, the assays differing mostly in the methods of separation of free from antibody-bound antigen. The methods of Egan et al.[23] and MacSween et al.[24] require no preliminary perchloric acid extraction of the serum, and utilize a double antibody technique. The assay described by Thompson et al.[25] and that of LoGerfo et al.[26] employ an initial perchloric acid extraction step. The assay of Thompson et al. utilizes a classical Farr precipitation for complexes while that of LoGerfo et al. involves the use of zirconyl phosphate gel for this purpose. This latter assay is the most widely used in the United States.

Using the LoGerfo et al. assay, normal plasma levels among healthy nonsmoking adults are below 2.6 ng/mℓ (97% of subjects), while levels in smokers tend to be higher, with 19% of smokers above this value.[27] Results in a large study with this method are summarized in Table 4. In general, circulating CEA values in malignant disease are higher in the presence of metastases than when disease is localized. Representative illustrations are given in Table 5.

At present, the most useful clinical role of CEA is in monitoring therapy and detecting residual disease, particularly in colo-rectal carcinomas. If plasma CEA is elevated preoperatively, total surgical extirpation of the tumor is followed by a fall of CEA levels to normal between the 2nd and 18th days.[5] Failure of the CEA levels to return to normal is indicative of subtotal excision or suspected metastatic disease, and the subsequent elevation of CEA levels after an initial return to normal frequently precedes clinical evidence of recurrent disease.[28] Similarly, it has been reported in breast carcinoma that patients with elevated postoperative levels have a higher recurrence rate than their counterparts with normal postoperative levels.[29,30] As with all tumor mark-

TABLE 4

Plasma CEA Values in Various Malignant Disease States

Condition	Number of patients	Elevated[a] (%)
Pancreatic carcinoma	55	91
Lung carcinoma	181	76
Colon-rectum carcinoma	544	72
Gastric carcinoma	79	61
Breast carcinoma	125	47
Leukemia	40	37
Malignant lymphoma	72	35
Sarcoma	38	31

[a] ≥ 2.6 ng/ml, Z-gel assay.

From Hansen, H. J., Snyder, J. J., and Miller, E., *Hum. Pathol.,* 5, 139, 1974. With permission.

TABLE 5

Plasma CEA Values in Different Stages of Various Malignant Disease

Tumor	Stage	Number of patients	Elevated CEA (%)
Carcinoma of the colon and rectum	Dukes A	48	42
	Dukes B	52	69
	Dukes C	38	71
	Metastatic	74	89
Bronchogenic carcinoma	Local NoMo	24	63
	Local N + Mo	6	83
	Metastatic	7	86
Carcinoma of breast	Local NoMo		
		69	32
	Local N + Mo		
	Metastatic	32	66
Carcinoma of prostate	Local	28	18
	Metastatic	13	54
Bladder carcinoma	Local	69	32
	Metastatic	24	33
Carcinoma of cervix	Stage 0	7	14
	Stage 1	14	36
	Stage 2	9	55
	Stage 3	9	55

From Laurence, D. J. R. and Neville, A. M., *Br. J. Cancer,* 26, 335, 1972. With permission.

ers, it should be stressed that normal values of CEA do not rule out recurrence or metastases.

Preoperative CEA levels are of some prognostic significance, with high levels correlating with a greater likelihood of recurrent disease and shorter disease free interval in colorectal carcinoma.[31] High CEA values have also been correlated with histological evidence of blood vessel, lymphatic or perineural invasion.[21]

As with AFP, the CEA assay has been found useful for following the relative tumor burden of patients being treated for metastatic disease. In both breast and colorectal carcinomas, elevated levels decrease in patients responding to therapy and increase again prior to or at the time of disease progression.[31-34] In addition, it has been suggested that patients with metastatic breast carcinoma and high CEA levels have a poorer prognosis than patients with normal or low values.[34]

A major drawback ot the CEA assay as currently performed is the relatively high prevalence of moderate elevations of CEA levels in a variety of nonmalignant diseases. This is particularly true of cirrhosis of the liver, gastric ulcers, granulomatous colitis, diverticulosis, pancreatitis, pneumonia, chronic renal disease, and emphysema.[5,26,27,35] Levels in such patients seldom exceed 20 ng/mℓ by the zirconyl phosphate gel assay, but overlap extensively with levels found in malignant disease, particularly in its early stages.

Attempts have therefore been made to improve the specificity of the CEA assay by further characterization of the immunoreactive species. Although a number of closely related molecules have been identified, they have yet to receive extensive clinical testing.[5,35-38] It seems clear that there is much yet to be learned about CEA, its purification, structure, function, clinical usefulness, and its relation to the substantial numbers of similar antigens, which have since been described.

IV. ALPHA$_2$H-GLOBULIN

Buffe et al.[39] immunized rabbits against fetal liver, producing an antibody which identified a glycoprotein with α_2 electrophoretic mobility. This substance was present as a monomer or dimer in normal adult liver and spleen, whereas more highly polymerized forms were found in the fetal liver and in certain tumors. Further, the amount of α_2 H-globulin present in the tumors was greater than that in the normal adult tissues.

Alpha$_2$ H-globulin shares many properties with ferritin (vide infra), but is reported to differ in solubility, sugar content, and the oxidation state of the iron content.[40] Although its normal metabolic role is unclear, it does appear to be immunosuppressive in vitro.[39]

The clinical application of circulating levels of α_2H-globulin has been investigated.[39,40] Levels in normal adult serum were found by radioimmunoprecipitation to be less than 150 ng/mℓ, while much higher levels were found in association with malignant disease (Table 6). The major nonmalignant condition associated with elevated levels was myocardial infarction. The prevalence of elevated α_2H-globulin levels in pediatric malignancy is summarized in Table 7. High circulating levels of α_2H-globulin were associated with a worse prognosis in leukemia,[41] and sequential values were of prognostic significance after surgical removal of solid tumors, with recurrence of elevated levels preceding clinical detection of tumor recurrences.[39,40]

V. FERRITINS

Ferritin, an iron storage protein, exists in various molecular forms consisting of hybrids of at least two dissimilar subunits. Immunologically, cross-reactive abnormal isoferritins have been detected in human and animal tumor cells.[42,43] Alpert et al.[44] found in human hepatoma an isoferritin corresponding to a fetal form absent from normal adult liver.

Halliday et al.[45] demonstrated tumor-specific isoferritins in the tumor tissue, but not the serum of four cancer patients; other studies have also documented elevated total circulating ferritin levels in association with a variety of tumors. Representative

TABLE 6

Serum α_2 H-globulin by Radioimmunodiffusion in Adult
Sera

Condition	Number tested	Levels > 200 ng/ml	
		Number	(%)
Healthy young adults	67	0	0
Myocardial infarction	103	82	80
Other severe disease	413	83	20
Tumor of:			
Liver	59	40	67.7
Stomach	38	22	57.8
Colon	42	23	54.7
Breast	54	28	51.8
ENT[a]	63	31	49.2
Lung	72	28	38.8
Other	168	82	48.8

[a] Oto-rhino-laryngology

From Buffe, D. and Rimbaut, C., *Ann. N.Y. Acad. Sci.,*
259, 417, 1975. With permission.

TABLE 7

Serum α_2 H-globulin by Radioimmunodiffusion in Sera of Children

Condition	Number tested	Levels > 200 ng/ml	
		Number	(%)
Healthy or benign disease	177	16	9
With malignant tumor	460	369	80
Tumor type:			
Hepatoma	49	45	91
Teratoma	43	22	51
Neuroblastoma	87	68	78
Nephroblastoma	88	77	87.5
Lymphoreticulosarcoma	35	30	85.7
Osteosarcoma	27	20	74
Embryonic sarcoma	41	33	80
Brain carcinoma	34	29	80
Other	56	45	80

From Buffe, D. and Rimbaut, C., *Ann. N.Y. Acad. Sci.,* 259, 417, 1975. With
permission.

data from a study by Mori et al.[46] is presented in Table 8. No information was presented concerning serial data with respect to relative tumor burden.

Marcus et al.[47] isolated an acidic isoferritin from breast tissue. Using a radioimmunoassay, elevated serum levels were detected in 14 of 38 patients with breast cancer prior to surgery as compared to 65 of 97 patients with metastatic disease, 0 of 117 normal women and 0 of 57 normal men, 22 of 73 patients with inflammatory diseases, and 18 of 31 patients with hematologic malignancies. In addition, it has been suggested

TABLE 8

Elevations of Serum Ferritin Detected by Countercurrent Immunoelectrophoresis

Disease state	Number of patients tested	Number of patients with elevated levels	Elevated (%)
Healthy controls	70	1	1.4
Blood bank donors	100	0	—
Collagen diseases	43	1	2.3
Pregnancy	15	1	6.7
Nonmalignant hematologic diseases	46	9	19.6
Other benign diseases	104	2	1.9
Malignancies			
Leukemias	100	54	54.0
Lymphoreticular	20	12	60.0
Multiple myeloma	47	11	23.4
Stomach cancer	19	8	42.1
Liver cancer	9	5	55.6
Rectal carcinoma	7	3	42.9
Lung carcinoma	9	2	22.2

From Mori, W., Asakawa, H., and Taguchi, T., *J. Natl. Cancer Inst.*, 55, 513, 1975. With permission.

that breast cancer patients with elevated preoperative serum ferritin levels have a poorer prognosis than patients with normal levels.[48]

VI. HUMAN CHORIONIC GONADOTROPIN (HCG)

Human chorionic gonadotropin (HCG) is a glycoprotein hormone normally produced in the syncytiotrophoblastic cells of the placenta.[49] Physicochemical heterogeneity among HCG molecules appears to be a reflection of varying sialic acid content.[50] The protein portion of the molecule consists of two noncovalently linked subunits, alpha and beta. The alpha subunit is cross reactive with analogous subunits of the pituitary glycoprotein tropic hormones, luteinizing hormone, follicle stimulating hormone, and thyroid stimulating hormone. Specificity is conferred by the beta subunit.

HCG is produced by a variety of trophoblastic and nontrophoblastic tumors in both sexes. The amino acid composition of such HCG is identical with the normal placental hormone, though the secretory rate is usually lower in tumor cells than in the placenta.[51]

Several radioimmunoassays for HCG are available.[52-54] Because of the cross reactivity of the alpha subunit with other glycoprotein hormones, assays directed to the HCG beta subunit have greater specificity than those directed to the intact molecule with alpha reactivity.[55]

Radioimmunoassay for the beta subunit of HCG reveals levels up to 2 ng/mℓ in serum of normal controls[56-58] possibly due to cross-reacting substances.[59] Serum levels in patients with various tumors are shown in Table 9. Elevated HCG levels are most prevalent in patients with testicular tumors and gestational trophoblastic disease; less frequently, high levels are found in patients with other tumors. Although not specific for HCG, assays directed at the glycoprotein hormones alpha subunit detected elevated levels in 14 of 28 (50%) patients with functioning islet cell carcinomas, as compared to beta subunit directed assays with elevations in 6 of 27 (22%) patients.[58]

Women with untreated gestational trophoblastic disease have uniformly elevated

TABLE 9

Prevalence of Elevated Levels of Immunoreactive HCG in Sera of Patients with Tumors[a]

Type of tumor	Number of patients	Number elevated	Elevated (%)
Gestational trophoblastic disease	49	49	100
Testicular:			
Embryonal	52	30	58
Seminoma	16	6	38
Teratocarcinoma	4	2	50
Choriocarcinoma	8	8	100
Unspecified	17	13	76
Leukemias	191	3	2
Myeloma	65	4	6
Lymphomas	251	5	2
Sarcomas	39	3	8
Lung	147	13	9
Ovarian	12	5	42
Breast	33	4	12
Melanoma	98	9	9
Alimentary tract	220	33	15
Pancreas	42	14	33
Liver	91	15	16

[a] Adapted from References 57, 60, 61.

HCG levels,[61] and sequential levels have proven to be an accurate measure of tumor response to therapy.[56,59,60,62] Immediately after chemotherapy, there is a transient rise in HCG levels which may reflect release of preformed HCG from damaged cells.[63]

Sequential HCG levels have in general correlated with clinical course in the nontrophoblastic tumors, although less accurately than is true of the trophoblastic tumors.[60,64,65]

VII. ALKALINE PHOSPHATASES

These glycoprotein isoenzymes are to some degree organ or tissue specific.[60] Normal human serum alkaline phosphatases originate in bone, biliary cells, intestine, and placenta.[66] Only the biliary and bone isoenzymes can be identified in most normal sera, but in 40%, the intestinal fraction is also present and correlates with blood group O secretor status.[66]

Elevated levels of the bone isoenzyme are found in patients with tumors metastatic to bone as well as with primary malignant bone tumors, particularly osteoblastic osteogenic sarcoma.[66] Lower levels are present in other primary malignant bone tumors. Hepatocellular carcinoma is not associated with an alkaline phosphatase elevation unless there is biliary obstruction or bile duct proliferation.[66]

The placental alkaline phosphatase (Regan) isoenzyme is normally present in the microvilli of the trophoblastic cells and is also found in the serum of women with gestational choriocarcinoma.[60] It is not present in fetal serum or the serum of normal men and nonpregnant women.[60] Distinguishing features from other alkaline phosphatases include inhibition by L-phenylalanine, but not by L-homoarginine.[67,68] Variants of the Regan isoenzyme have been described, particularly the Nagao variant, which, although immunologically identical, is inhibited not only by L-phenylalanine, but also

TABLE 10

Prevalence of Elevated Levels of Placental Alkaline Phosphatase (Regan Isoenzyme)[a]

	Number Patients	Number (%) Elevated
Nonmalignant disease — Total	81	9 (11)
Hepatitis	6	0
Cirrhosis	8	2 (25)
Ulcerative colitis	4	2 (50)
Other GI disease	7	1
Peripheral vascular disease	7	3 (43)
Miscellaneous	49	1
Malignant Diseases		
Carcinoma of:		
Lung	51	7 (4)
Breast	49	6 (12)
Colon	53	5 (9)
Ovary	23	5 (22)
Cervix	93	14 (15)
Prostate	8	1
Lymphoma/leukemia	68	3 (4)
Sarcomas	22	3 (14)
Normal subjects	139	5 (4)

[a] Adapted after References 70, 71.

by L-leucine, L-isoleucine, L-valine and EDTA.[69] The prevalence of elevated levels of the Regan isoenzyme in various conditions is summarized in Table 10. As with other circulating markers, it may be of value in individual cases in whom elevated levels are detected at the onset of treatment, but its prevalence in nonmalignant conditions renders its use as a unique diagnostic test in cancer screening dubious.

VIII. ACID PHOSPHATASE

From seven to eight isoenzymes of acid phosphatase are present in different tissues of the body.[72,73] Isoenzymes number 2 and 4 are characteristic of prostatic carcinoma. Several enzyme assays are available, but a recently described radioimmunoassay appears to be more sensitive than the conventional enzyme assays.[74] In some patients, a normal value for total serum or plasma acid phosphatase may be present, but the isoenzyme pattern may be abnormal.[72] Representative results are reproduced in Table 11. Elevated levels were found more frequently in advanced than in localized prostatic cancer, and were also present in a small percentage of other types of cancer and in benign prostatic disease. Elevation of acid phosphatase following prostatic massage is transient, unless renal function is impaired.[72] Elevated levels of the enzyme appear to be useful for following the tumor burden during treatment.[72]

IX. OTHER ENZYMES

Lactic dehydrogenase (LDH) exists in five isoenzymic forms, which are made up of varying combinations of two basic polypeptide subunits. Total serum LDH is elevated in approximately 40% of cancer patients, and an abnormal isoenzyme pattern is found in 51%.[66] The most common situation is simultaneous elevation of all five isoenzymes, seen particularly in leukemias and lymphomas, but also in benign conditions involving

TABLE 11

Percentage of Patients with Elevated Prostatic Acid Phosphatase in Serum as Detected by Radioimmunoassay and by Enzyme Assay

Group	Number of patients	Elevation by Radioimmunoassay				Elevation by Enzyme Assay above 0.2 Sigma U/1.0 mℓ	
		above 6.6 ng/0.1 mℓ		above 8.0 ng/0.1 mℓ			
		Number	(%)	Number	(%)	Number	(%)
Normal controls	50	0	0	0	0	0	0
Prostatic Cancer							
Stage I	24	12	50	8	33	3	12
Stage II	33	26	79	26	79	5	15
Stage III	31	25	81	22	71	9	29
Stage IV	25	24	96	23	92	15	60
Benign prostatic hyperplasia	36	5	14	2	6	0	0
Total prostatectomy	28	5	18	1	4	0	0
Other cancer	83	14	17	9	11	7	8
Gastrointestinal disorders	20	2	10	1	5	0	0

Modified from Foti, A. G., Cooper, J. F., Herschman, H., and Malvaez, R. R., *N. Engl. J. Med.*, 297, 1357, 1977. With permission.

hemolysis and in pernicious anemia. Solitary elevation of isoenzyme LDH$_5$, the normal liver isoenzyme, may occur even in the absence of liver metastases. Finally, elevation of LDH$_1$, and LDH$_2$ may be seen, a pattern which resembles the elevation characteristic of myocardial infarction. The use of LDH isoenzymes for following the therapy of malignant disease has not been shown to be particularly useful in clinical practice.

Aldolase catalyzes the metabolism of fructose-1,6-diphosphate (FDP) and fructose-1-phosphate (FIP). Isoenzymes characteristic of different normal tissues exhibit differing ratios of affinity for these two substrates; a FDP to FIP ratio of 54 is characteristic of the skeletal muscle isoenzyme, and 1.0 for the liver isoenzyme.[66] Normal human serum aldolase shows an FDP to FIP ratio of 2.8 ± 0.4, and elevated levels of this ratio have been described in patients with a variety of tumors with or without hepatic metastases.

Arylsulfatase B is one of a group of enzymes widely distributed in human tissue. It has been found in human urine in association with a number of carcinomas.[75] In particular, the prevalence of elevated urinary values has been correlated with the stage of disease in colorectal cancer, varying from 12% in Duke's A to 81% in Duke's D, and changes in the urinary levels tended to follow the clinical course of the disease.[76]

Elevated levels of ribonuclease in human serum have been associated with ovarian carcinoma,[77] prostatic carcinoma,[73] and myeloma, as well as benign conditions including toxic goiter, cardiac, hepatic, and renal failure.[78]

X. FETAL SULPHOGLYCOPROTEIN ANTIGEN (FSA)

Sulphoglycoproteins histochemically similar to those appearing during human fetal gastrointestinal development have been demonstrated in gastric cancer cells, and a similar substance has been isolated from the gastric juice of patients with gastric carcinoma.[79] The molecule also contains antigenic determinants cross reactive with blood group substances and with carcinoembryonic antigen. It is present in the gastric juice of about 96% of patients with gastric carcinoma, 14% of patients with peptic ulceration and in from 3 to 7% of the normal population.[5,79] The role of this antigen in sequential follow-up of patients following resection of gastric carcinoma is limited, since it tends to persist despite adequate surgery.[5]

XI. POLYAMINES

The following low molecular weight aliphatic polyamines have been identified in humans and studied as possible circulating cancer markers:

Putrescine	$H_2H - (CH_2)_4 - NH_2$
Spermidine	$H_2N - (CH_2)_4 - NH - (CH_2)_3 - NH_2$
Spermine	$H_2N - (CH_2)_3 - NH - (CH_2)_4 - NH - (CH_2)_3 - NH_2$
Cadaverine	$H_2N - (CH_2)_5 - NH_2$

Crystals of spermine phosphates were first found in human serum by van Leeuwenhuek in 1678. Spermine was rediscovered by Ladenburg and Abel in 1888. They have been the subject of several recent reviews.[80-87] They are found in all types of prokaryotic and eukaryotic cells as well as in viruses; recent studies indicate that they may play fundamental roles in various cellular replicative processes.

Putrescine is synthesized in animal cells by the decarboxylation of L-ornithine. Putrescine is then the precursor for the formation of spermidine and spermine. It is condensed with an aminopropyl group from 5-adenosylmethylthiopropylamine, a decarboxylation product of S-adenosylmethionine. Spermine results from the addition of another aminopropyl group to spermidine with the donor again being decarboxylated S-adenosylmethionine; the enzyme is spermine synthetase. In animal cells, ornithine decarboxylase is the rate-limiting enzyme for polyamine synthesis; its reaction product, putrescine, is necessary for spermidine synthesis and can also activate the other rate-limiting enzyme, S-adenosylmethionine decarboxylase. Cadaverine is apparently formed from the decarboxylation of lysine.

Various methods have been used to detect and quantitate polyamines in tissues and body fluids and have been recently reviewed.[85,86] Of the various procedures, enzymatic and paper electrophoresis have the lowest sensitivity (3000 to 5000 pmol). Radioimmunoassay and gas chromatography using electron capture detectors to determine polyamines as their pentafluorobenzoyl derivatives appear to have the greatest sensitivity (1 pmol). The use of high pressure amino acid analyzer and high pressure liquid or gas chromatography permit detection of intermediate quantities (down to 25 pmol) within 30 min. Of these analytical approaches, the radioimmunoassay using a rabbit antispermine antibody is probably the least specific due to cross reactions with other polyamines; however, it does appear to permit estimation of total polyamine amounts in human serum.[88]

Multiple studies in experimental tumors have suggested a link between carcinogenesis and the activation of polyamine synthesis. In addition, polyamines are present in tumors in relatively high concentrations, though it is not completely clear whether they exist as free bases or complexed with other substances.[80-86]

In 1971, Russell[89] reported that patients with various types of cancer excreted polyamines in their urine. It was also demonstrated that polyamines may be excreted as conjugates which yield the free chemical after hydrolysis. It was observed that elevation of urinary polyamines was not specific for any particular type of cancer, but was

TABLE 12

Prevalence of Elevated Polyamine Levels in Selected Diseases[a]

Disease State	Putrescine		Spermidine		Spermine	
	Number Elevated/ Number Studied	(%)	Number Elevated/ Number Studied	(%)	Number Elevated/ Number Studied	(%)
Nonmalignant diseases	28/104	(27)	26/104	(25)	13/104	(12)
Lung carcinoma	14/82	(50)	41/82	(50)	28/82	(34)
Breast carcinoma	2/84	(2)	24/84	(28)	21/84	(25)
Colon carcinoma	28/90	(31)	39/90	(43)	59/90	(66)
Pancreatic carcinoma	8/29	(28)	7/29	(24)	9/29	(31)
Gastric carcinoma	5/24	(21)	3/24	(12)	7/24	(29)
Melanoma	3/25	(12)	8/24	(33)	6/25	(24)
Burkitt's lymphoma	6/7	(86)	7/7	(100)	7/7	(100)

[a] Adapted from References 91, 92.

present in almost all patients with tumors prior to therapy.[90] Surgical removal of a portion of the tumor or medical treatment that resulted in a remission in leukemia patients was associated with reduction in the urinary level of polyamines.[89,90]

Waalkes et al.[91] in 1975 reported urinary polyamine levels in tumor patients, patients with other diseases, and normal controls (Table 12). An automated ion exchange method was used to determine the values of putrescine, spermidine, spermine, and cadaverine. They found a distinct sex difference in the mean level of urinary putrescine and to a lesser extent spermine. Females without disease excreted greater amounts of putrescine than males, but males excreted greater amounts of spermine than females. In females, there was a decrease in the average level of putrescine excretion with increasing age, but this did not apply to males. Children excreted greater amounts than adults on a body-weight basis. The polyamine levels were not affected by diet and remained in a narrow range for any one individual at different time intervals. It was found that patients with diseases other than malignancy may excrete greater amounts of polyamines than normals. In these patients, the greatest incidence of elevation above 2 SD of the normal mean was found for putrescine (27%), next highest for spermidine (22%), and the least for spermine (13%).

In tumor patients, there was a wide variation in the proportion of patients with polyamine elevations about 2 SD in different tumor types. Almost 50% of the patients with bronchogenic carcinoma had elevated levels of putrescine and spermidine while 34% had elevated levels of spermine. For colon carcinoma patients, 31% had elevated putrescine levels, 43% elevated spermidine levels, and 66% elevated spermine levels. A later report showed that in patients with metastatic breast carcinoma, 14% had elevated putrescine levels, 11% elevated spermidine levels, and 1% elevated spermine levels.[92] Patients with liver metastases had a higher incidence of elevated spermine levels than patients without liver metastases, independent of tumor type. The highest levels and greatest frequency of elevated polyamine levels were found in patients with Burkitt's lymphoma.[93] Changes in the polyamine levels reflected response to therapy in Burkitt's lymphoma[93] and in breast carcinoma.[94]

Elevated cadaverine levels were found in a variety of different malignancies, but at a lower frequency than for the other polyamines, though occasionally cadaverine was the only polyamine elevated.[91,94]

It was concluded from these studies that increased polyamine excretion is not tumor specific and that many patients with cancer may have normal values. It was suggested that following polyamine levels may be helpful in assessing disease status in patients with Burkitt's lymphoma, colon cancer, bronchogenic carcinoma, and in those breast carcinoma patients with initially elevated values.

Dreyfuss et al.[95] also studied urinary excretion of polyamines and demonstrated elevated values in 37 of 42 (88%) cancer patients. There were also elevated values in 24 of 54 (44%) patients with nonmalignant disease, especially infections. Elevated levels of all three polyamines, putrescine, spermidine, and spermine, simultaneously, were almost exclusively seen in patients with malignancy.

Lipton et al.[96] examined putrescine, spermidine, and spermine levels in the urine of patients with metastatic malignancies and found that 38 of 56 patients had two or more levels elevated greater than 2 SD above the normal range. The histologic type of tumor and the sites of metastatic involvement did not appear to influence the urinary polyamine levels. In this study, breast cancer patients were not as likely to have elevated levels as other adenocarcinomas. Six patients with localized tumor all had elevated values. In a larger series of localized tumors, 24 of 26 patients had two or more elevated urinary polyamines.[97] Some patients with various nonmalignant conditions also had elevated values, and it was felt that the total urinary polyamine level and elevations of two or more individual polyamines were the most reliable guide to the presence of malignancy.

Townsend et al.[98] studied patients with malignant melanoma and found that there were more frequent elevations of two or more urinary polyamine levels in patients with disseminated melanoma at a time of active progression than in patients with localized stable disease. Both mean values and percentages of patients with elevated values increased as stage, activity, or both, increased. This study indicated that urinary polyamines may be useful for following the impact of therapy in this particular tumor if conditions which falsely elevate levels can be identified and eliminated.

Elevated urinary polyamines have also been found in lymphosarcoma, Hodgkin's disease, acute myelocytic leukemia,[85] and prostate carcinoma.[99] In the latter study, there was a higher incidence of elevated polyamines with the more histologically malignant prostatic tumors.

Mean urinary putrescine, spermidine, and spermine levels have been reported to all be significantly increased with hematological and solid malignancies as compared to normals.[100,101] In patients with multiple myeloma, putrescine levels were correlated with clinical activity of the disease and the in vitro labeling index of marrow plasma cells. Spermidine values were felt to reflect tumor cell burden, and serial studies showing a greater than twofold rise in urinary spermidine levels during treatment were correlated with cell kill and later clinical response. In 17 patients, the serum and urine polyamine levels were found to be comparable. It was concluded that baseline polyamine values reflected tumor cell mass and growth fraction and cell kill was indicated by an early increase in blood or urine spermidine levels during treatment.

Nishioka and Romsdahl[102] found serum polyamine levels elevated above the normal means in patients with colorectal and breast carcinomas as well as sarcomas, melanomas, and Hodgkin's disease. Serum spermidine showed a higher than normal mean in 75% of specimens.

Bachrach[85] also found high levels of polyamines in the serum of a majority of cancer patients. Effects of treatment were studied in patients with multiple myeloma and embryonal cell carcinoma. There were elevated levels of putrescine and spermidine immediately after the initiation of chemotherapy, but these decreased if a remission occurred. These and other studies[100] suggest that an initial increase in serum polyamines may indicate effective therapy. These results correlate with rat models in which serum spermidine levels initially increased if a tumor regression occurred after the initiation of therapy.[103,104]

Marten et al.[105,106] found that there were elevated levels of putrescine and spermidine in the cerebrospinal fluid (CSF) of most patients with central nervous system tumors when compared to the CSF of patients with nonmalignant central nervous system disorders. Patients with glioblastomas and medulloblastomas had the highest values. Effective treatment reduced the levels to those of the nontumor patient reference group. The concentration in the CSF was not related to the CSF protein concentration and the authors concluded that the polyamine levels in the CSF did not reflect alterations in the blood brain barrier, but might relate to tumor burden.

XII. NUCLEOSIDES

The primary nucleosides that have been investigated as potential circulating biological markers are pseudouridine (Ψ), N^2,N^2-dimethylguanosine (m_2^2G), and 1-methylinosine (m^1I). These nucleosides are found predominantly in transfer ribonucleic acid (tRNA) and to a much lesser extent in ribosomal RNA.[107,108] Following degradation of tRNA, the free Ψ is excreted intact and not reincorporated into tRNA; thus its excretion is considered to reflect tRNA turnover.[109,110] The methylated tRNA bases are synthesized after the synthesis of the tRNA molecule by specific methyl transferases using S-adenosylmethionine as the methyl group donor.[111-114] Upon degradation of tRNA, the methylated nucleosides are presumably not reincorporated into RNA so that their presence in urine is evidence of the extent of tRNA modification and rate of turnover.[115,116]

It has been suggested that aberrant nucleic acid methylation is related to malignant transformation.[117] The group of tRNA methyl transferases show both qualitative and quantitative changes in systems undergoing shifts in regulatory processes.[118-120] Increased tRNA methylase activity has been found in extracts of malignant tumors as compared to normal tissue.[120-122] Also, the rRNAs from both animal and human tumors have been reported to contain elevated amounts of specific methylated nucleic acid bases.[122]

Using a radioimmunoassay to measure serum levels of m_2^2G and Ψ, Levine et al.[123] found a high proportion of patients with acute leukemia, breast cancer, and other malignancies to have elevated serum levels.

Waalkes et al.[124] used gas-liquid chromatography to measure levels of m_2^2G, m^1I, and Ψ in urine. A large percentage of patients with various malignancies had excretion levels elevated above two standard deviations from the normal (Table 13). In general, for any given patient, if one of the nucleosides was found elevated in the urine, the levels for one or both of the others were usually increased. To a greater degree than Ψ or m^1I, m_2^2G was more frequently elevated. Of 62 patients with disease other than cancer, Ψ was elevated in one patient, m_2^2G in 12 patients, and m^1I in 13 patients. It was not determined in this study if serial measurements of these nucleosides would be useful in following the patient's clinical course, but other studies have suggested that they may be in selected patients.[94] Increased urinary excretion of 7-methylguanine, 1-methylguanine, N^2-dimethylguanine, 1-methylhypoxanthine, and adenine in hepatoma patients compared to normals and to patients with cirrhosis of the liver has also been reported.[125]

XIII. HYDROXYPROLINE

Hydroxyproline is a nonessential amino acid that comprises 13% of the amino acid

TABLE 13

Prevalence of Elevated Nucleosides in Patients

Disease State	m$_2^2$G Number Elevated/ Number Tested	(%)	m^{1}I Number Elevated/ Number Tested	(%)	Ψ Number Elevated/ Number Tested	(%)
Nonmalignant diseases	12/62	(19)	13/62	(21)	1/62	(2)
Lung carcinoma	38/57	(67)	37/57	(65)	17/59	(29)
Colon carcinoma	27/43	(63)	29/48	(60)	24/49	(49)
Other gastrointestinal tumors	17/30	(57)	19/35	(54)	13/38	(34)
Breast carcinoma	36/69	(52)	30/72	(42)	21/74	(28)
Melanoma	9/13	(69)	8/13	(62)	6/13	(46)
Miscellaneous other tumors	16/30	(53)	19/40	(48)	17/46	(37)

Adapted from Waalkes, T. P., Gehrke, C. W., Zumwalt, R. W., Chang, S. Y., Lakings, D. B., Tormey, D. C., Ahmann, D. L., and Moertel, C. G., *Cancer (Philadelphia)*, 36, 390, 1975. With permission.

content of collagen and is almost absent in other tissue proteins.[126] Collagen degradation provides the major source of hydroxyproline in urine.[127-129] It is excreted in free and bound form in human urine. The free form normally makes up about 4% of the total and the bound form can be released from its polypeptide by acid hydrolysis. The urinary excretion of hydroxyproline is mainly derived from the degradation of newly synthesized (soluble) collagen. Only 5 to 10% of the hydroxyproline released into the circulation is excreted in the urine; the rest is metabolized. Thus, relatively large changes in collagen degradation must occur to alter the rate of urinary excretion of hydroxyproline, but increases are associated with disorders of bone, including acromegaly, hyperthyroidism, hyperparathyroidism, Paget's disease, Marfan's syndrome, Hurler's syndrome, malabsorption with secondary osteomalacia, and rheumatoid arthritis.[130-137] Studies have also shown increased hydroxyproline excretion in patients with radiologically demonstrable metastases in bone. Elevation of urinary hydroxyproline occurs with both osteolytic and osteoblastic lesions.[138,139] The urinary hydroxyproline to creatinine (HOP to Cr) ratio was reported to correlate better with radiologically demonstrable bony metastases than did the absolute 24-hr urinary hydroxyproline excretion.[140] Patients were kept on a diet low in hydroxyproline containing foods during the urine collection. Powles et al.[141] have recently shown that an early morning ½-hr fasting urine sample is just as accurate as the 24-hr specimen and is not affected as much by dietary factors. Patients who develop bony metastases have been shown to have elevated HOP to Cr ratios which preceded X-ray and clinical evidence of metastases by 1 to 7 months.[140]

Elevation of serum alkaline phosphatase had not been found to correlate with the presence of bone metastases as well as the HOP to Cr ratio and was not as sensitive in predicting the development of bony lesions.[140] Bone scans may detect lesions as early as does urinary hydroxyproline, but when a bone scan is not diagnostic or there may be osteoporosis or spondylosis, the measurement of hydroxyproline may provide supporting evidence for the presence of bone metastases.[142]

Sequential hydroxyproline excretion measurements have been reported to give information on the activity of bone metastases and response to treatment earlier than Xrays or bone scan.[142] The prognostic role of HOP to Cr ratios is uncertain. Gielen et al.[142] did not find a correlation between hydroxyproline excretion levels and prognosis. However, in a study by Cuschieri,[143] patients with breast cancer who had elevated urinary hydroxyproline excretion at the time of disease presentation had a higher failure rate over a 5-year follow-up than did women with normal urinary levels.

XIV. OTHER MARKERS AND APPROACHES

As noted in the introduction to this chapter, a variety of molecules have received attention as potential cancer markers. For the most part, the information on these substances is fragmentary. Nevertheless, it is noteworthy that a variety of serum-protein endgroup carbohydrates may be useful in following the course of various diseases, especially breast carcinoma.[144-147] Also of interest are the reports suggesting a similar role in lung and breast carcinomas for serum calcitonin levels.[148,149] Of course, the utility of calcitonin measurements in the diagnosis and follow-up of medullary thyroid carcinoma is a classical example of a very useful marker.[150,151]

Due to the difficulties in finding a highly specific circulating marker for malignancy, investigators working with breast cancer populations have turned to measuring multiple marker levels in an attempt to increase detection sensitivities.[92,152,153] With such an approach, using breast cancer as the model, one group has reported the detection of abnormalities in 99% of patients with metastatic disease, 69% of preoperative patients, and 54% of postoperative patients.[154] In that study, simultaneous measurement of three tRNA nucleosides, the polyamines, HCG, and CEA were utilized. A preliminary report has suggested that the sequential analysis of multiple markers may be of clinical value for following the relative tumor burden of individual patients.[155]

XV. SUMMARY AND CONCLUSIONS

From the foregoing, it is evident that no ideal tumor markers have yet been discovered. With all of the available substances, a compromise must be reached between under-interpretation with its attendant lack of sensitivity and over-interpretation which, because of the frequent tumor marker elevations associated with nonmalignant diseases, will lead to over-diagnosis.

There exist, nonetheless, many situations in which tumor markers are clinically valuable. Most of these pertain to the detection of postsurgical recurrent disease, or the monitoring of response to various therapeutic modalities. In addition, certain markers may be of ancillary diagnostic value, particularly acid phosphatase in prostatic carcinoma, HCG in choriocarcinoma, calcitonin in medullary thyroid carcinoma, and markers such as CEA or AFP which, when highly elevated, may be useful in distinguishing between nonmalignant disease and advanced cancer. Future research must concentrate on the delineation of more highly specific tumor markers, as well as the relative value of early therapeutic intervention for recurrences diagnosed solely on the basis of marker elevations.

REFERENCES

1. Abelev, G. I., Perova, S. D., Khramkova, Z. A., Postnikova, Z. A., and Irlin, I. S., Production of embryonal α-globulin by transplantable mouse hepatomas, *Transplantation*, 1, 174, 1963.
2. Tatarinov, Yu. S., Content of embryo-specific α-globulin in fetal and neonatal sera and sera from adult humans with primary carcinoma of the liver, *Vopr. Med. Khim.*, 2, 20, 1965.

3. **Bergstrand, C. G. and Czar, B.**, Demonstration of a new protein fraction in serum from the human fetus, *Scand. J. Clin. Lab. Invest.*, 8, 174, 1956.

4. **Pick, A. I., Shoenfeld, Y., Schreibman, S., Weiss, H., and Ben-Bassat, M.**, Alpha-fetoprotein assay. Significance and clinical applications, *N.Y. State J. Med.*, 75, 1403, 1975.

5. **Laurence, D. J. R. and Neville, A. M.**, Foetal antigens and their role in the diagnosis and clinical management of human neoplasms: a review, *Br. J. Cancer*, 26, 335, 1972.

6. **Cowchock, F. S. and Jackson, L. G.**, Diagnostic use of maternal serum alpha-fetoprotein levels, *Obstet. Gynecol.*, 47, 63, 1976.

7. **Brock, D. J. H.**, The prenatal diagnosis of neural tube defects, *Obstet. Gynecol. Surv.*, 31, 32, 1976.

8. **Waldmann, T. A. and McIntire, K. R.**, The use of radioimmunoassay for users of RIA for alpha-fetoprotein in the diagnosis of malignancy, *Cancer (Philadelphia)*, 34, 1510, 1974.

9. **Franchimont, P., Zangerle, P. F., Debruche, M. L., Proyard, J., Simon, M., and Gaspard, U.**, Radioimmunoassay of alpha-fetoprotein in various normal and pathologic conditions, *Ann. Biol. Clin. (Paris)*, 33, 139, 1975.

10. **Tsuchida, Y., Endo, Y., Urano, Y., and Ishida, M.**, α-fetoprotein in yolk sac tumor, *Ann. N. Y. Acad. Sci.*, 259, 221, 1975.

11. **Nørgaard-Pedersen, B., Albrechtsen, R., and Teilum, G.**, Serum alpha-foetoprotein as a marker for endodermal sinus tumour (yolk sac tumour) or a vitelline component of 'teratocarcinoma,' *Acta Path. Microbiol. Scand. Sect. A*, 83, 573, 1975.

12. **Cohen, H., Starkovsky, N., and Olweney, C.**, Alpha-fetoprotein in urine of hepatoma patients, *Lancet*, 2, 717, 1975.

13. **Tonami, N., Aburano, T., and Hisada, K.**, Comparison of alpha fetoprotein radioimmunoassay method and liver scanning for detecting primary hepatic cell carcinoma, *Cancer (Philadelphia)*, 36, 466, 1975.

14. **Endo, Y. and Kanai, K.**, The clinical significance of α-fetoprotein, *Jpn. J. Clin. Pathol.*, 23, 356, 1975.

15. **McIntire, K. R., Vogel, C. L., Primack, A., Waldmann, T. A., and Kyalwazi, S. K.**, Effect of surgical and chemotherapeutic treatment on alpha-fetoprotein levels in patients with hepatocellular carcinoma, *Cancer (Philadelphia)*, 37, 677, 1976.

16. **Borgeaux, C., Martel, N., Sizaret, P., and Guerrin, J.**, Prognostic value of alpha-fetoprotein radioimmunoassay in surgically treated patients with embryonal cell carcinoma of the testis, *Cancer (Philadelphia)*, 38, 1658, 1976.

17. **Gold, P. and Freedman, S. O.**, Demonstration of tumor-specific antigens in human colonic carcinomata by immunological and absorption techniques, *J. Exp. Med.*, 121, 439, 1965.

18. **Terry, W. D., Henkart, P. A., Coligan, J. E., and Todd, C. W.**, Carcinoembryonic antigen: characterization and clinical applications, *Transplant. Rev.*, 20, 100, 1974.

19. **Coligan, J. E., Lautenschleger, J. T., Egan, M. L., and Todd, C. W.**, Isolation and characterization of CEA, *Immunochemistry*, 9, 377, 1972.

20. **Gold, P.**, Embryonic origin of human tumor-specific antigens, *Progr. Exp. Tumor Res.*, 14, 43, 1971.

21. **Martin, F., Martin, M. S., and Bourgeaux, C.**, Fetal antigens in human digestive tumors, *Eur. J. Cancer*, 12, 165, 1976.

22. **Shuster, J., Silverman, M., and Gold, P.**, Metabolism of human carcinoembryonic antigen in xenogeneic animals, *Cancer Res.*, 33, 65, 1973.

23. **Egan, M. L., Lautenschleger, J. T., Coligan, J. E., and Todd, C. W.**, Radioimmunoassay of carcinoembryonic antigen, *Immunochemistry*, 9, 289, 1972.

24. **MacSween, J. M., Warner, N. L., Bankhurst, A. D., and Mackay, I. R.**, Carcinoembryonic antigen in whole serum, *Br. J. Cancer*, 26, 356, 1972.

25. **Thompson, D. M. P., Krupey, J., Freedman, S. O., and Gold, P.**, The radioimmunoassay of circulating carcinoembryonic antigen of the human digestive system, *Proc. Natl. Acad. Sci. U.S.A.*, 64, 161, 1969.

26. **LoGerfo, P. L., Krupey, J., and Hansen, H. J.**, Demonstration of an antigen common to several varieties of neoplasia. Assay using zirconyl phosphate gel, *N. Engl. J. Med.*, 285, 138, 1971.

27. **Hansen, H. J., Snyder, J. J., and Miller, E.**, Carcinoembryonic antigen (CEA) assay: a laboratory adjunct in the diagnosis and management of cancer, *Hum. Pathol.*, 5, 139, 1974.

28. **Mach, J.-P., Jaeger, Ph., Bertholet, M.-M., Ruegsegger, C.-H., Loosli, R. M., and Pettavel, J.**, Detection of recurrence of large-bowel carcinoma by radioimmunoassay of circulating carcinoembryonic antigen (C.E.A.), *Lancet*, 2, 535, 1974.

29. **Wang, D. Y., Bulbrook, R. D., Hayward, J. L., Hendrick, J. C., and Franchimont, P.**, Relationship between plasma carcinoembryonic antigen and prognosis in women with breast cancer, *Eur. J. Cancer*, 11, 615, 1975.

30. **Myers, R. E., Sutherland, D. J. A., Meakin, W., and Malkin, D.G.,** Prognostic value of CEA in breast cancer patients, *Proc. Am. Assoc. Cancer Res.,* 19, 148, 1978.

31. **Holyoke, E. D., Chu, T. M., and Murphy, G. P.,** CEA as a monitor of gastrointestinal malignancy, *Cancer (Philadelphia),* 35, 830, 1975.

32. **Skarin, A. T., Delwiche, R., Zamcheck, N., Lokich, J. J., and Frei, E., III,** Carcinoembryonic antigen: clinical correlation with chemotherapy for metastatic gastrointestinal cancer, *Cancer (Philadelphia),* 33, 1239, 1974.

33. **Steward, A. M., Nixon, D., Zamcheck, N., and Aisenberg, A.,** Carcinoembryonic antigen in breast cancer patients — serum levels and disease progress, *Cancer (Philadelphia),* 33, 1246, 1974.

34. **Tormey, D. C., Waalkes, T. P., Snyder, J. J., and Simon, R. M.,** Biological markers in breast carcinoma. III. Clinical correlations with carcinoembryonic antigen, *Cancer (Philadelphia),* 39, 2397, 1976.

35. **Lamerz, R. and Fateh-Moghadam, A.,** Oncofetal antigens. II. Carcinoembryonic antigen (CEA), *Klin. Wochenschr.,* 53, 193, 1975.

36. **Edgington, T. S., Astarita, R. W., and Plow, E. F.,** Association of an isomeric species of carcinoembryonic antigen with neoplasia of the gastrointestinal tract, *N. Engl. J. Med.,* 293, 103, 1975.

37. **Burtin, P., Chavanel, G., and Hirsch-Marie, H.,** Characterization of a second normal range antigen that cross-reacts with CEA, *J. Immunol.,* 111, 1926, 1973.

38. **Martin, E. W., Jr., Kibbey, W. E., DiVecchia, L., Anderson, G., Catalano, P., and Minton, J. P.,** Carcinoembryonic antigen, clinical and historical aspects, *Cancer (Philadelphia),* 37, 62, 1976.

39. **Buffe, D. and Rimbaut, C.,** α_2-H-Globulin, a hepatic glycoferroprotein: characterization and clinical significance, *Ann. N.Y. Acad. Sci.,* 259, 417, 1975.

40. **Yachi, A., Akahonai, Y., Takahashi, A., and Wada, T.,** Clinical significance of α_2H-globulin, *Ann. N.Y. Acad. Sci.,* 259, 435, 1975.

41. **Martin, J. P., Charlionnet, R., and Ropartz, C.,** L' α_2H sérique au cours des hémopathies malignes et des cirrhoses, Valeur évolutive, *Presse Med.,* 79, 2313, 1971.

42. **Drysdale, J. W. and Singer, R. M.,** Carcinofetal human isoferritins in placenta and HeLa cells, *Cancer Res.,* 34, 3352, 1974.

43. **Drysdale, J. W. and Alpert, E.,** Carcinofetal human isoferritins, *Ann. N.Y. Acad. Sci.,* 259, 427, 1975.

44. **Alpert, E., Coston, R. L., and Drysdale, J. W.,** Carcinofetal human liver ferritins, *Nature (London),* 242, 194, 1973.

45. **Halliday, J. W., McKeering, L. V., and Powell, L. W.,** Isoferritin composition of tissues and serum in human cancers, *Cancer Res.,* 36, 4486, 1976.

46. **Mori, W., Asakawa, H., and Taguchi, T.,** Antiserum against leukemia cell ferritin as a diagnostic tool for malignant neoplasms, *J. Natl. Cancer Inst.,* 55, 513, 1975.

47. **Marcus, D. M., and Zinberg, N.,** Measurement of serum ferritin by radioimmunoassay: results in normal individuals and patients with breast cancer, *J. Natl. Cancer Inst.,* 55, 791, 1975.

48. **Jacobs, A., Jones, B., Ricketts, C., Bulbrook, R. D., and Wang, D. Y.,** Serum ferritin concentration in early breast cancer, *Br. J. Cancer,* 34, 286, 1976.

49. **Canfield, R. E., Morgan, F. J., Kammerman, S., Bell, J. J., and Agosto, G. M.,** Studies of human chorionic gonadotropin, *Recent Progr. Horm., Res.,* 27, 121, 1971.

50. **Wiese, H. C., Graesslin, D., and Braendle, W.,** Microheterogeneity of HCG reflected in the β-subunits, *Acta Endocrinol. (Copenhagen), Suppl.,* 173, 55, 1973.

51. **Braunstein, G. D., Grodin, J. M., Vaitukaitis, J., and Ross, G. T.,** Secretory rates of human chorionic gonadotropin by normal trophoblast, *Am. J. Obstet. Gynecol.,* 115, 447, 1973.

52. **Vaitukaitis, J. L., Braunstein, G. D., and Ross, G. T.,** A radioimmunoassay which specifically measures human chorionic gonadotropin in the presence of human luteinizing hormone, *Am. J. Obstet. Gynecol.,* 113, 751, 1972.

53. **Kosasa, T. S., Levesque, L. A., Goldstein, D. P., and Taynor, M. L.,** Clinical use of a solid-phase radioimmunoassay specific for human chorionic gonadotropin, *Am. J. Obstet. Gynecol.,* 119, 784, 1974.

54. **Kardana, A. and Bagshawe, K. D.,** A rapid, sensitive and specific radioimmunoassay for human chorionic gonadotropin, *J. Immunol. Methods,* 9, 297, 1976.

55. **Arends, J.,** Non-identical reaction of undissociated HCG and HCG-β subunit with anti-HCGβ serum, *Acta Endocrinol. (Copenhagen),* 80, 374, 1975.

56. **Jones, W. B., Lehr, M., and Lewis, J. L., Jr.,** Radioimmunoassay of the β-subunit of human chorionic gonadotropin, monitor of chemotherapy in gestational trophoblastic neoplasm, *Surg. Forum,* 563, 1973.

57. **Braunstein, G. D., Vaitukaitis, J. L., Carbone, P. P., and Ross, G. T.,** Ectopic production of human chorionic gonadotropin by neoplasms, *Ann. Int. Med.,* 78, 39, 1973.

58. Kahn, C. R., Rosen, S. W., Weintraub, B. D., Fajans, S. S., and wgorden, P., Ectopic production of chorionic gonadotropin and its subunits by islet-cell tumors. A specific marker for malignancy, *N. Engl. J. Med.*, 297, 565, 1977.

59. Tomoda, Y., Asai, Y., Arii, Y., Kaseki, S., Nishi, H., Miwa, T., Saiki, N., and Ishizuka, N., Criteria of complete remission from trophoblastic neoplasia with the use of human chorionic gonadotropin (HCG) excretion pattern as a parameter, *Cancer (Philadelphia)*, 40, 1016, 1977.

60. Rosen, S. W., Weintraub, B. D., Vaitukaitis, J. L., Sussman, H. H., Hershman, J. M., and Muggia, F. M., Placental proteins and their subunits as tumor markers, *Ann. Int. Med.*, 82, 71, 1975.

61. Vaitukaitis, J. L., Human chorionic gonadotropin as a tumor marker, *Ann. Clin. Lab. Sci.*, 4, 276, 1974.

62. Goldstein, D. P., Pastorfide, G. B., Osathanondh, P., and Kosasa, T. S., A rapid solid phase radioimmunoassay specific for human chorionic gonadotropin in gestational trophoblastic disease, *Obstet. Gynecol.*, 45, 527, 1975.

63. Hussa, R. O., Pattillo, R. A., Delfs, E., and Mattingly, R. F., Actinomycin D stimulation of HCG production by human choriocarcinoma, *Obstet. Gynecol.*, 42, 651, 1973.

64. Muggia, F. M., Rosen, S. W., Weintraub, B. D., and Hansen, H. H., Ectopic placental proteins in nontrophoblastic tumors. Serial measurements following chemotherapy, *Cancer (Philadelphia)*, 36, 1327, 1975.

65. Tormey, D. C., Waalkes, T. P., and Simon, R. M., Biological markers in breast carcinoma. II. Clinical correlations with human chorionic gonadotrophin, *Cancer (Philadelphia)*, 39, 2391, 1977.

66. Reynoso, G., Biochemical tests in cancer diagnosis, in *Cancer Medicine*, Holland, J. F., and Frei, E., III, Eds., Lea & Febiger, Philadelphia, 1973, 335.

67. Watanabe, K. and Fishman, W. H., Application of the stereospecific inhibitor L-phenylalanine to the enzymology of intestine alkaline phosphatase, *J. Histochem. Cytochem.*, 12, 252, 1964.

68. Rufo, M. B., and Fishman, W. H., L-homoarginine, a specific inhibitor of liver type alkaline phosphatase, applied to the recognition of liver type enzyme activity in rat intestine, *J. Histochem. Cytochem.* 20, 336, 1972.

69. Fishman, W. H., Perspectives on alkaline phosphatase isoenzymes, *Am. J. Med.*, 56, 617, 1974.

70. Nathanson, L. and Fishman, W. H., New observations on the Regan isoenzyme of alkaline phosphatase in cancer patients, *Cancer (Philadelphia)*, 27, 1388, 1971.

71. Usategui-Gomez, M., Yeager, F. M., and de Castro, A. F., Regan isoenzyme in normal human sera, *Cancer Res.*, 34, 2544, 1974.

72. Yam, L. T., Clinical significance of the human acid phosphatases. A review, *Am. J. Med.*, 56, 604, 1974.

73. Chu, T. M., Wang, M. C., Kuciel, R., Valenzula, L., and Murphy, G. P., Enzyme markers in human prostatic carcinoma, *Cancer Treat. Rep.*, 61, 193, 1977.

74. Foti, A. G., Cooper, J. F., Herschman, H., and Malvaez, R. R., Detection of prostatic cancer by solid-phase radioimmunoassay of serum prostatic acid phosphatase, *N. Engl. J. Med.*, 297, 1357, 1977.

75. Dzialoszynski, L. M., The clinical value of arylsulfatase estimation in urine, *Clin. Chim. Acta*, 2, 542, 1957.

76. Morgan, L. R., Samuels, M. S., Thomas, W., Krementz, E. T., and Meeker, W., Arysulfatase B in colorectal cancer, *Cancer (Philadelphia)*, 36, 2337, 1975.

77. Sheid, B., Lu, T., Pedrinan, L., and Nelson, J. H., Jr., Plasma ribonuclease. A marker for the detection of ovarian cancer, *Cancer (Philadelphia)*, 39, 2204, 1977.

78. Chretien, P. B., Matthews, W., Jr., and Twomey, P. L., Serum ribonucleases in cancer: relation to tumor histology, *Cancer (Philadelphia)*, 31, 175, 1973.

79. Häkkinen, I. P. T., A population screening for fetal sulfoglycoprotein antigen in gastric juice, *Cancer Res.*, 34, 3069, 1974.

80. Bachrach, U., Metabolism and function of spermine and related compounds, *Ann. Rev. Microbiol.*, 24, 109, 1970.

81. Cohen, S.S., *Introduction to the Polyamines*, Prentice-Hall, Englewood Cliffs, N. J., 1971.

82. Russell, D. H., Polyamines in growth-normal and neoplastic, in *Polyamines in Normal and Neoplastic Growth*, Russell, D. H., Ed., Raven Press, N.Y., 1973, 1.

83. Bachrach, U., *Function of Naturally Occurring Polyamines*, Academic Press, New York, 1973.

84. Takeda, Y. and Inoue, H., Polyamines and multiplication of cells, *Horumon To Rinsho*, 23, 111, 1975.

85. Bachrach, U., Polyamines as chemical markers of malignancy, *Ital. J. Biochem.*, 25, 77, 1976.

86. Cohen, S. S., Conference on polyamines in cancer, *Cancer Res.*, 37, 939, 1977.

87. Tabor, H. and Tabor, C. W., Biosynthesis and metabolism of 1,4 diaminobutane, spermidine, spermine and related amines, in *Adv. Enzymol. Relat. Areas Mol. Biol.*, 36, 203, 1972.

88. **Bartos, D., Campbell, R. A., Bartos, F., and Grettie, D. P.,** Direct determination of polyamines in human serum by radioimmunoassay, *Cancer Res.,* 35, 2056, 1975.

89. **Russell, D. H.** Increased polyamine concentration in the urine of human cancer patients, *Nature (London), New Biol.,* 233, 144, 1971.

90. **Marton, L. J., Vaughn, J. G., Hawk, I. A., Levy, C. C., and Russell, D. H.,** Elevated polyamine levels in serum and urine of cancer patients: detection by a rapid automated technique utilizing an amino acid analyzer. In *Polyamines in Normal and Neoplastic Growth,* Russell, D. H., Ed., Raven Press, N.Y., 1973, 367.

91. **Waalkes, T. P., Gehrke, C. W., Tormey, D. C., Zumwalt, R. W., Hueser, J. N., Kuo, K. C., Lakings, D. B., Ahmann, D. L., and Moertel, C. G.,** Urinary excretion of polyamines by patients with advanced malignancy, *Cancer Chemother. Rep.,* 59, 1103, 1975.

92. **Tormey, D. C., Waalkes, T. P., Ahmann, D., Gehrke, C. W., Zumwalt, R. W., Snyder, J., and Hansen, H.,** Biologic markers in breast carcinoma. I. Incidence of abnormalities of CEA, HCG, three polyamines and three minor nucleosides, *Cancer (Philadelphia),* 35, 1095, 1975.

93. **Waalkes, T. P., Gehrke, C. W., Bleyer, W. A., Zumwalt, R. W., Olweny, C. L. M., Kuo, K. C., Lakings, D. B., and Jacobs, S. A.,** Potential biologic markers in Burkitt's lymphoma, *Cancer Chemother. Rep.,* 59, 721, 1975.

94. **Tormey, D. C. and Waalkes, T. P.,** Biochemical markers in cancer of the breast, *Recent Results Cancer Res.,* 57, 78, 1976.

95. **Dreyfuss, F., Chayen, R., Dreyfuss, G., Dvir, R., and Ratan, J.,** Polyamine excretion in the urine of cancer patients, *Isr. J. Med. Sci.,* 11, 785, 1975.

96. **Lipton, A., Sheehan, L. M., and Kessler, G. F., Jr.,** Urinary polyamine levels in human cancer, *Cancer (Philadelphia),* 35, 464, 1975.

97. **Lipton, A., Sheehan, L., Mortel, R., and Harvey, H. A.,** Urinary polyamine levels in patients with localized malignancy, *Cancer (Philadelphia),* 38, 1344, 1976.

98. **Townsend, R. M., Bandu, P. W., and Marton, L. J.,** Polyamines in malignant melanoma. Urinary excretion and disease progress, *Cancer (Philadelphia),* 38, 2088, 1976.

99. **Fair, W. R., Wehner, N., and Brorsson, U.,** Urinary polyamine levels in the diagnosis of carcinoma of the prostate, *J. Urol.,* 114, 88, 1975.

100. **Durie, B. G. M., Salmon, S. E., and Russell, D. H.,** Polyamines as markers of response and disease activity in cancer chemotherapy, *Cancer Res.,* 37, 214, 1977.

101. **Russell, D. H., Durie, B. G. M., and Salmon, S. E.,** Polyamines as predictors of success and failure in cancer chemotherapy, *Lancet,* 2, 797, 1975.

102. **Nishioka, K. and Romsdahl, M. M.,** Elevation of putrescine and spermidine in sera of patients with solid tumors, *Clin. Chim. Acta,* 57, 155, 1974.

103. **Russell, D. H., Gullino, P. M., Marton, L. J.,and leGendre, S. M.,** Polyamine depletion of the MTW9 mammary tumor and subsequent elevation of spermidine in the sera of tumor-bearing rats as a biochemical marker of tumor regression, *Cancer Res.,* 34, 2378, 1974.

104. **Russell, D. H., Looney, W. B., Kovacs, C. J., Hopkins, H. A., Marton, L. J., leGendre, S.M., and Morris, H. P.,** Polyamine depletion of tumor tissue and subsequent elevation of spermidine in the sera of rats with 3924A hepatomas after 5-fluorouracil administration, *Cancer Res.,* 34, 2382, 1974.

105. **Marton, L. J., Heby, O., and Wilson, C. B.,** Increased polyamine concentrations in the cerebrospinal fluid of patients with brain tumors, *Int. J. Cancer,* 14, 731, 1974.

106. **Marton, L. J., Heby, O., Levin, V. A., Lubich, W. P., Crafts, D. C., and Wilson, C.B.,** The relationship of polyamines in cerebrospinal fluid to the presence of central nervous system tumors, *Cancer Res.,* 36, 973, 1976.

107. **Dunn, D. B.,** Additional components in ribonucleic acid of rat-liver fractions, *Biochem. Biophys. Acta,* 34, 286, 1959.

108. **Hall, R. H.,** A general procedure for the isolation of "minor" nucleosides from ribonucleic acid hydrolysates, *Biochemistry,* 4, 661, 1965.

109. **Weissman, S. M., Eisen, A. Z., Lewis, M. and Karon, M.,** Pseudouridine metabolism — III. Studies with isotopically labeled pseudouridine, *J. Lab. Clin. Med.,* 60, 40, 1962.

110. **Dlugajczyk, A. and Eiler, J. J.,** Lack of catabolism of 5-ribosyluracil in man, *Nature (London),* 212, 611, 1966.

111. **Biswas, B. A., Edmonds, M., and Abrams, R.,** The methylation of the purines of soluble ribonucleic acid with methyl labeled methionine, *Biochem. Biophys. Res. Commun.,* 6, 146, 1961.

112. **Fleissner, E. and Borek, E.,** Studies on the enzymatic methylation of soluble RNA. I. Methylation of the S-RNA polymer, *Biochemistry,* 2, 560, 1963.

113. **Srinivasan, P. R. and Borek, E.,** The species variation of RNA methylase, *Proc. Natl. Acad. Sci.*

114. **Sharma, O. K., Kerr, S. J., Lipshitz-Wiesner, R., and Borek, E.,** Regulation of the tRNA methylases, *Fed. Proc.,* 30, 167, 1971.

115. **Dlugajcyk, A. and Eiler, J. J.**, Studies on 5-riboeyluracil in man, *Proc. Soc. Exp. Biol. Med.*, 123, 453, 1966.

116. **Borek, E., Baliga, B. S., Gehrke, C. W., Kuo, K. C., Belman, S., Troll, W., and Waalkes, T. P.**, High turnover rate of transfer RNA in tumor tissue, *Cancer Res.*, 37, 3362, 1977.

117. **Gantt, R. R.**, Is aberrant nucleic acid methylation related to malignant transformation?, *J. Natl. Cancer Inst.*, 53, 1505, 1974.

118. **Sharma, O. K. and Borek, E.**, A mechanism of estrogen action on gene expression at the level of translation, *Cancer Res.*, 36, 4320, 1976.

119. **Riddick, D. H. and Gallo, R. C.**, Correlation of transfer RNA methylase activity with growth and differentiation in normal and neoplastic tissues, *Cancer Res.*, 30, 2484, 1970.

120. **Waalkes, T. P., Adamson, R. H., O'Gara, R. W., and Gallo, R. C.**, Transfer RNA methylase activity in normal monkey liver and in carcinogen-induced hepatoma, *Cancer Res.*, 31, 1069, 1971.

121. **Tsutsui, E., Srinivasan, P. R., and Borek, E.**, t-RNA methylases in tumors of animal and human origin, *Proc. Natl. Acad. Sci., U.S.A.*, 56, 1003, 1966.

122. **Borek, E.**, Introduction to symposium: tRNA and tRNA modification in differentiation and neoplasia, *Cancer Res.*, 31, 596, 1971.

123. **Levine, L., Waalkes, T. P. and Stolbach, L.**, Serum levels of N^2,N^2-dimethylguanosine and pseudouridine as determined by radioimmunoassay for patients with malignancy, *J. Natl. Cancer Inst.*, 54, 341, 1975.

124. **Waalkes, T. P., Gehrke, C. W., Zumwalt, R. W., Chang, S. Y., Lakings, D. B., Tormey, D.C., Ahmann, D. L., and Moertel, C. G.**, The urinary excretion of nucleosides of ribonucleic acid by patients with advanced cancer, *Cancer (Philadelphia)*, 36, 390, 1975.

125. **Ho, Y. and Lin, H. J.**, Patterns of excretion of methylated purines in hepatocellular carcinoma, *Cancer Res.*, 34, 986, 1974.

126. **Stein, W. H. and Miller, E. G., Jr.**, The composition of elastin, *J. Biol. Chem.*, 125, 599, 1938.

127. **Lindsedt, S. and Prockop, D. J.**, Isotopic studies on urinary hydroxyproline as evidence for rapidly catabolized forms of collagen in the young rat, *J. Biol. Chem.*, 236, 1399, 1961.

128. **Prockop, D. J.**, Isotopic studies on collagen degradation and the urine excretion of hydroxyproline, *J. Clin. Invest.*, 43, 453, 1964.

129. **Kivirikko, K. I., Laitinen, O., Lamberg, B.-A.**, Value of urine and serum hydroxyproline in the diagnosis of thyroid disease, *J. Clin. Endocrinol. Metab.*, 25, 1347, 1965.

130. **Ziff, M., Kibrick, A., Dresner, E., and Gribetz, H. J.**, Excretion of hydroxyproline in patients with rheumatic and non-rheumatic diseases, *J. Clin. Invest.*, 35, 579, 1956.

131. **Prockop, D. J. and Sjoerdsma, A.**, Significance of urinary hydroxyproline in man, *J. Clin. Invest.*, 40, 843, 1961.

132. **Jasin, H. E., Fink, C. W., Wise, W., and Ziff, M.**, Relationship between urinary hydroxyproline and growth, *J. Clin. Invest.*, 41, 1928, 1962.

133. **Dull, T. A. and Henneman, P. H.**, Urinary hydroxyproline as an index of collagen turnover in bone, *N. Engl. J. Med.*, 268, 132, 1963.

134. **Keiser, H. R., Gill, J. R., Sjoerdsma, A., and Bartter, F. C.**, Relation between urinary hydroxyproline and parathyroid function, *J. Clin. Invest.*, 43, 1073, 1964.

135. **Crabbe, P. and Isselbacher, K. J.**, Urinary hydroxyproline excretion in malabsorption states, *Gastroenterology*, 48, 307, 1965.

136. **Kivirikko, K.I., Laitinen, O., Aer, J., and Halme, J.**, Studies with ^{14}C-proline on the action of cortisone on the metabolism of collagen in the rat, *Biochem. Pharmacol.*, 14, 1445, 1965.

137. **Nakagawa, M. and Tamaki, T.**, Urinary hydroxyproline excretion in orthopedic disease, *Nagoya J. Med. Sci.*, 27, 228, 1965.

138. **Platt, W. D., Doolittle, L. H., and Hartshorn, J. W. S.**, Urinary hydroxyproline excretion in metastatic cancer of bone, *N. Engl. J. Med.*, 271, 287, 1964.

139. **Hosley, H. F., Taft, E. G., Olson, K. B., Gates, S., and Beebe, R. T.**, Hydroxyproline excretion in malignant neoplastic disease, *Arch. Intern. Med.*, 118, 565, 1966.

140. **Guzzo, C. E., Pachas, W. M., Pinals, R. S., and Krant, M. J.**, Urinary hydroxyproline excretion in patients with cancer, *Cancer (Philadelphia)*, 24, 382, 1969.

141. **Powles, T. J., Dip, G. R. F., Leese, C. L., and Bondy, P. K.**, Early morning hydroxyproline excretion in patients with breast cancer, *Cancer (Philadelphia)*, 38, 2564, 1976.

142. **Gielen, F., Dequeker, J., Drochmans, A., Wildiers, J., and Merlevede, M.**, Relevance of hydroxyproline excretion to bone metastases in breast cancer, *Br. J. Cancer*, 34, 279, 1976.

143. **Cuschieri, A.**, Urinary hydroxyproline excretion and survival in cancer of the breast, *Clin. Oncol.*, 1, 127, 1975.

144. **Rosato, F. E., Seltzer, M., Mullen, J. and Rosato, E. F.**, Serum fucose in the diagnosis of breast cancer, *Cancer (Philadelphia)*, 28, 1575, 1971.

145. Evans, A. S., Dolan, M. F., Sobocinski, P. X., and Quinn, F. A., Utility of serum protein-bound neutral hexoses and L-fucose for estimation of malignant tumor extension and evaluation of efficacy of therapy, *Cancer Res.*, 34, 538, 1974.

146. Mrochek, J. E., Dinsmore, S. R., Tormey, D. C., and Waalkes, T. P., Protein-bound carbohydrates in breast cancer. Liquid-chromatographic analysis for mannose, galactose, fucose and sialic acid in serum, *Clin. Chem.*, 22, 1516, 1976.

147. Waalkes, T. P., Gehrke, C. W., Tormey, D. C., Woo, K. B., Kuo, K. C., Snyder, J., and Hansen, H., Biologic markers in breast carcinoma. IV. Serum fucose-protein ratio; comparisons with carcinoembryonic antigen and human chorionic gonadotropin, *Cancer (Philadelphia)*, 41, 1871, 1978.

148. Coombes, R. C., Hillyard, C. J., Greenberg, P. B., and MacIntyre, I., Plasma immunoreactive calcitonin in patients with non-thyroid tumours, *Lancet*, 1, 1080, 1974.

149. Coombes, R. C., Easty, G. C., Detre, S. I., Hillyard, C. J., Stevens, U., Gingis, S. I., Galante, L. S., Heywood, L., MacIntyre, I., and Neville, A. M., Secretion of immunoreactive calcitonin by human breast carcinomas, *Br. Med. J.*, 4, 197, 1975.

150. Wolfe, H. J., Melvin, K. E. W., Cervi-Skinner, S. J., Al Saadi, A. A., Juliar, J. F., Jackson, C. E., and Tashjian, A. H., Jr., C-cell hyperplasia preceding medullary thyroid carcinoma, *N. Engl. J. Med.*, 289, 437, 1973.

151. Goltzman, D., Potts, J. T., Jr., Ridgway, E. C., and Maloof, F., Calcitonin as a tumor marker. Use of the radioimmunoassay for calcitonin in the postoperative evaluation of patients with medullary thyroid carcinoma, *N. Engl. J. Med.*, 290, 1035, 1974.

152. Franchimont, P., Zangerle, P. F., Nogarede, J., Bury, J., Molter, F., Reuter, A., Hendrick, J. C., and Collette, J., Simultaneous assays of cancer-associated antigens in various neoplastic disorders, *Cancer (Philadelphia)*, 38, 2287, 1976.

153. Coombes, R. C., Powles, T. J., Gazet, J. C., Ford, H. T., Nash, A. G., Sloane, J. P., Hillyard, C. J., Thomas, P., Keyser, J. W., Marcus, D., Zinberg, N., Stimson, W. H., and Neville, A. M., A biochemical approach to the staging of human breast cancer, *Cancer (Philadelphia*, 40, 937, 1977.

154. Tormey, D. C. and Waalkes, T. P., Clinical correlation between CEA and breast cancer, *Cancer (Philadelphia)*, 42, 1507, 1978.

155. Woo, K. B., Waalkes, T. P., Ahmann, D.L., Tormey, D. C., Gehrke, C. W., and Oliverio, V. T., A quantitative approach to determining disease response during therapy using multiple biologic markers: applications to carcinoma of the breast, *Cancer (Philadelphia)*, 41, 1685, 1978.

INDEX